General Surgery Residency Survival Guide

Asanthi Ratnasekera • Marc Neff
Kahyun Yoon-Flannery • Alec Beekley
Editors

General Surgery Residency Survival Guide

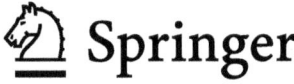 Springer

Editors
Asanthi Ratnasekera
Division of Trauma and Surgical Critical
Care and Acute Care Surgery
Christiana Care Health System
Newark, DE, USA

Kahyun Yoon-Flannery
Janet Knowles Breast Cancer Center
MD Anderson Cancer Center
at Cooper and Cooper Medical School
of Rowan University
Camden, NJ, USA

Marc Neff
Center for Surgical Weight Loss
Jefferson Health of New Jersey
Cherry Hill, NJ, USA

Alec Beekley
Jefferson Comprehensive Weight
Management
Thomas Jefferson University Hospital
Philadelphia, PA, USA

ISBN 978-3-031-25616-5   ISBN 978-3-031-25617-2   (eBook)
https://doi.org/10.1007/978-3-031-25617-2

This Springer imprint is published by the registered company Springer Nature Switzerland AG
The registered company address is: Gewerbestrasse 11, 6330 Cham, Switzerland

Preface

As the editors, we are proud to introduce this book to all surgical residents and medical students interested in a career as a surgeon. We, as surgeons of various specialties, have struggled through the many years of intensive work hours, administrative duties, and clinical expectations to complete a surgical residency. We relied on mentors, colleagues, and many trial-by-fire experiences to survive. We acknowledge that it was not the best way to learn. It is even more of a challenge for trainees today.

There are roughly 260 surgical residencies in the United States. Most residents experience variable degrees of shock and awe once they start on their very first day. The demands of residency are very high, and most residents are ill-prepared. The current overall dropout rate is approximately 16%. There is much evidence for higher burnout rates, suicide rates, addiction, and divorce rates amongst all surgeons compared to other medical and nonmedical careers. The COVID-19 pandemic has further elucidated the lack of preparedness of surgical residents for the challenges of a surgical residency. There is a critical need for education and guidance on surviving this challenging portion of their career. Unfortunately, the experiences of trial and error are the basis for survival. Resiliency training is often overlooked as part of the traditional surgical training. This has to change.

This book is founded on many conversations with general surgery residents during these past 2 years. We aim to utilize the experiences of current residents at several residency programs, covering a wide variety of topics, with variable experiences based on differing ages, races, sexes, and marital statuses. We hope that it serves as a guide and resource to help residents and medical students prepare for the rigors of surgical residency. Information contained would hopefully help residents and students to not only survive but also thrive. We hope that this book will serve to fill the void in resiliency training.

Although many commercial products, tools, and programs are mentioned in the chapters, we have received no financial agreements or funds for the publication of this book.

Best of luck to all of you in your future surgical careers!

Newark, DE, USA   Asanthi Ratnasekera
Cherry Hill, NJ, USA   Marc Neff
Camden, NJ, USA   Kahyun Yoon-Flannery
Philadelphia, PA, USA   Alec Beekley

Contents

Part II   Clinical Duties

Part III   Life Outside of Work/Finances

Part I
Academics

Chapter 1
Mentorship: How to Spot a Good Mentor and Hold on Tight

Brian M. Till and Shale Mack

Introduction

Mentorship takes many forms, and most surgical residents will have multiple senior surgeons that they recognize as mentors during their training. Some of these individuals will provide clinical mentorship, others will serve as research mentors, and still others may help a trainee shape the kind of work-life balance they seek to obtain. In the academic literature, an important distinction is made between mentorship and sponsorship, with sponsors recognized as well-respected individuals in the community whom put forward more junior persons for specific opportunities [1]. This chapter focuses on mentorship.

Seeking a Mentor

It is critical to identify potential mentors early in one's training. We recommend looking to recent graduates from your program pursuing career trajectories similar to that you hope to follow and finding out who their mentors were. This can often be achieved by reviewing publications from various current residents and recent graduates at the institution where you are training. Once you have identified a potential

B. M. Till (✉)
Thomas Jefferson University Hospitals, Philadelphia, PA, USA
e-mail: Brian.Till@jefferson.edu

S. Mack
Sidney Kimmel Medical College at Thomas Jefferson University, Philadelphia, PA, USA
e-mail: Shale.Mack@students.jefferson.edu

© The Author(s), under exclusive license to Springer Nature Switzerland AG 2023
A. Ratnasekera et al. (eds.), *General Surgery Residency Survival Guide*,
https://doi.org/10.1007/978-3-031-25617-2_1

mentor, we recommend you reach out to former mentees. This step helps one learn more about a potential mentor, their strengths, and tips for developing and maintaining a successful relationship with this surgeon. If seeking a research mentor, we recommend carefully studying the potential mentor's previous research to better understand the type of work they conduct (basic science, outcomes research, etc.); understand the datasets they use and skills needed to successfully perform this research; understand the type of group they work with to conduct research (be it division partners, bench scientists, statisticians, clinical trial experts, etc.); understand the overall narrative of the work; and understand their typical annual volume of publications. Understanding these factors can help you to recognize how you may fit into the mentor's research.

Developing a Strong Working Relationship

Mutual benefit is key to a strong mentor-mentee relationship. For residents, the potential benefits are clear: to gain skills, to build a network within a future specialty or subspecialty of interest, and to potentially make a meaningful personal connection. Mentees often fail to appreciate that they, too, bring benefits to the mentor-mentee relationship and that, as their skill set grows, their capacity to provide value for their mentor increases. Indeed, at many institutions, faculty involvement as mentors and the achievements of their mentees are required in applications for academic advancement. Mentees can increase faculty productivity, broaden the skill sets and capabilities of the mentor's research, and even—one day—become potential partners or collaborators.

To develop a strong relationship, we recommend a mentee (1) identify the skill set they bring to collaboration and (2) define how they hope to broaden that skill set by working with a particular mentor. Mentees should not undervalue their existing skills. For example, the capabilities to draft a meaningful manuscript, provide high-quality literature review, and manage a submission process are important skills.

Critical to this is a mutual understanding and development of shared goals. Considering a mentor's goals can help a mentee appreciate joint collaboration on a new level. These goals might include advancing within a professional society or moving up the academic ladder within an institution. We recommend consistent and directive goal setting (semesterly vs. quarterly), including targeting specific conference deadlines and project completion timelines.

Furthermore, it is important that a potential mentor and mentee be transparent about their constraints. For the resident, time constraints may arise in January as the American Board of Surgery In-Training Examination (ABSITE) approaches or on weekends due to childcare limitations or call schedules. Mentors may be limited by clinical duties if partners are out on leave or there are changes to the hospital system. Identifying these constraints early, articulating them, and setting appropriate goals for productivity are key. In doing so, hurdles can be tackled as adjustments to plans rather than setbacks.

Maintaining a Strong Working Relationship

Set the relationship up for success with easy wins early. Whether collaborating on book chapters, case reports, or invited commentaries, select projects that are likely to result in quick wins. Success breeds success, and these achievements can lay the foundation for the collaboration before taking on more challenging work, like in-depth quality improvement projects, prospective research, or large database studies. As time progresses, adapt your goals and stay hungry for more wins.

It is critical to meet consistently with a mentor in a setting where disruptions are limited. For example, try to avoid meeting immediately before or after an operative case. This may require flexibility on the mentee's part, but meeting consistently is critical to advancing projects. If you run into trouble or need direction, this is your time to ask. Every meeting should have an agenda, and the mentee should seek to share new data or drafts along with the proposed agenda several days before a meeting. Also include in the agenda status updates of ongoing projects and focused action items. We additionally recommend creating a shared Gantt chart (Fig. 1.1) in which each project can be tracked.

Celebrate successes, no matter how small. Getting a project to the point of submission should be recognized as wins, as should be timely grant submissions, regardless of whether these works are accepted or funded. Invitations for revision are regarded as very important wins, as nearly all editorial boards that offer a revision intend to publish a manuscript if authors are able to rigorously respond to the critiques. Abstract acceptances, manuscript publications, and awards—these, too, should be celebrated by the research group writ large.

Broader project	Sub-project	People responsible	Stakeholder/ organization	What does finished look like? (GOAL)	What does minimal deliverable look like?	Outstanding questions	6 Month Plan						2017
							Aug	Sept	Oct	Nov	Dec	Jan 2017	

Fig. 1.1 Gantt chart, which may be used to easily track projects

Dealing with Challenges in the Relationship

It is easy for a mentor-mentee relationship to become strained. When problems arise, we recommend identifying them early, speaking to the sources of the underlying strain dispassionately, and approaching a mentor with proposed solutions. Such problems may include increased clinical demands limiting the time in which a mentor can meet; a lack of available resources precluding the completion of a project; or larger-than-expected demands on a mentee's time that limits their productivity. In these cases, mature, candid proposals from the mentee for possible steps forward can help to improve the relationship and its productivity. In these instances, scaling work back to less time-consuming projects may be an answer. Alternatively, a mentee may consider the benefit of broadening the team, whether by looking for additional help from within the home university or by enlisting medical students. By finding potential solutions and bringing them to a mentor, a mentee can demonstrate both their creativity and dedication to the work. In cases of overextended mentors, we also recommend doing everything possible to reduce the workload for a mentor. Such steps can include drafting research-related emails or editorial board letters, managing submissions in journal portals, and meeting the mentor when available (i.e., being on call to connect on a weekend morning after an attending finishes rounding, for instance) if no other time allows.

Pearls
- Developing a strong mentor-mentee relationship can not only help boost your academic development, but also shape life goals and expand your network.
- In order to build such a relationship, be the mentee you would want: be profoundly enthusiastic, under-promise, and over-deliver.
- To the extent residency allows, be available, affable, and able.
- Always meet deadlines.
- Over time, success breeds success.
- Express appreciation for the time and energy your mentor is investing in you.

Reference

1. Ayyala MS, Skarupski K, Bodurtha JN, et al. Mentorship is not enough: exploring sponsorship and its role in career advancement in academic medicine. Acad Med. 2019;94(1):94–100. https://doi.org/10.1097/ACM.0000000000002398.

Chapter 2
ABSITE and the Boards: A Marathon Mindset

Walker Lyons and Emily Isch

Introduction

Standardized testing remains a part of a career in medicine. For surgery, there are a number of different tests you will have to take during and shortly after your residency. This chapter focuses on the tests run by the American Board of Surgery (ABS), including the annual American Board of Surgery In-Training Examination (ABSITE) and the two tests required to become board-certified in general surgery—the Qualifying Exam (QE) and the Certifying Exam (CE). These tests are more commonly referred to as the written and oral boards.

One of the most important things that residents can do to set themselves up for success with ABSITE and the boards is to take a long-term approach in preparing for them. While there are "study periods" leading up to the exams, these should not be viewed as tests that you can prepare for in a month or two. Instead, view your entire 5-year residency as a way to prepare for the boards, with the yearly ABSITE as a gauge on this preparation. By doing this, you will be better prepared for the exams, less stressed, and a more knowledgeable resident as reflected on the wards and in the operating room. Below we will focus on ways to do this within the busy schedule of residency and then focus on specifics for preparing for the written ABSITE and QE exams and the oral CE.

W. Lyons (✉) · E. Isch
Thomas Jefferson University Hospitals, Philadelphia, PA, USA
e-mail: Emily.Isch@jefferson.edu

© The Author(s), under exclusive license to Springer Nature Switzerland AG 2023
A. Ratnasekera et al. (eds.), *General Surgery Residency Survival Guide*,
https://doi.org/10.1007/978-3-031-25617-2_2

9

Reading Plan

Every resident should choose one core textbook and develop a reading plan. Historically, these have included Cameron's, Sabiston's, or Schwartz's, though others exist [1–3]. The book you choose is less important than picking one and developing a plan. A good reading plan should allow you to complete the entire textbook 1–2 times throughout your residency. Additionally, the best way to utilize this reading is a focused approach with taking notes, so that when the time comes to review the material for ABSITE or boards, it is readily available. It is important to be realistic when developing this plan; reading two pages of Cameron's every day (approximately 20 min or less of focused reading) will allow you to finish it twice partway through the fifth year of residency. Developing this habit early in residency will pay dividends throughout. And just like any habit (diet, exercise, sleep), know that you can fall off the wagon. While there are some days (or weeks!) where there will not be enough time for any reading due to your work schedule or life events, that does not mean you have failed; the faster you get back on the wagon, the better. This core reading will provide an important foundation for your surgical knowledge. The online SCORE curriculum can provide a framework with which you can organize your topic review or book chapters, with the option for accompanying/relevant questions each week [4].

ABSITE/Qualifying Exam

Both the ABSITE and QE are multiple choice examinations. The best way to directly prepare for these tests is with practice questions. Doing around ten questions a week is a good goal during the year. Closer to the test, set aside a dedicated study period to ramp up the number of questions per day. There are several different question banks with different strengths and weaknesses (Table 2.1). Over the course of a residency, expect to utilize a number of these question banks, as their educational value decreases once you have worked through a question bank more than one time. The

Table 2.1 Commonly used question banks for ABSITE and Qualifying Exam

Question bank	Comments
ABSITE Quest	Great mobile app, short, quick questions useful for building the habit of doing daily questions
SCORE	Questions are most like those found on ABSITE, utility of explanations varies based on question and author
SESAP®	More difficult questions that are better suited for senior residents preparing for QE
TrueLearn	Similar to UWorld with great answer explanations; questions can be too focused on minutia

content in SESAP® offered by the American College of Surgeons is often considered the most similar to the QE; therefore, it is beneficial to save this question bank until the fourth or fifth year of residency for dedicated QE studying.

In addition to question banks, it is also helpful to have a study text geared specifically towards the tests. *Behind The Knife* has become a staple for many residents over the past decade. The podcast has dedicated episodes geared towards the ABSITE and QE, broken down by topic [5]. Listening to these is great while commuting to work, exercising, or doing chores. The podcast creators have recently released a companion book that gives visual learners a text version to follow along with the podcast [6]. Another well-known text is *The ABSITE Review*, which covers similar information presented in bullet format [7].

The breakdown of the content on the exams can be found on the ABS website, which is useful in helping to prioritize which topics to study (https://www.absurgery.org/xfer/GS-ITE.pdf). Additionally, every year you will receive your ABSITE results, with a complete breakdown of percent correct by topic. Make a point to review material and questions on the topics that were a weakness before the next ABSITE or your QE.

Certifying Exam

The CE, or oral boards, is different than most of the tests you will have taken in your education up to this point. As an oral examination, it presents with a different set of skills than residents have developed through the countless written tests. It still requires the core knowledge you should be developing over your residency, which is why a reading plan is a crucial part to being successful. Additionally, finding a procedural textbook during residency is mandatory to being prepared for the operating room and will be useful for reviewing technical steps when preparing for your CE.

While expensive, taking a review course is recommended. Table 2.2 shows the different courses; explore the different options they offer, and pick the style that most suits your preferred learning method. Having a review textbook geared towards the CE can be beneficial as well. Table 2.3 shows different options. Again, this is a different type of test, so you will need resources to teach you the test-taking skills necessary to be successful on the CE.

Table 2.2 Review courses for the Certifying Exam

Course name	Website
Odyssey	http://www.surgery-board-review.com/index.html
The Osler Institution	https://www.osler.org/general-surgery/
The Pass Machine	https://www.thepassmachine.com/general-surgery-certifying-board-review/

Table 2.3 Review textbooks for the Certifying Exam	Book title
	Clinical Scenarios in Surgery [8]
	How to Win: On the American Board of Surgery Certifying Exam [9]
	Passing the General Surgery Oral Board Exam [10]
	Safe Answers for the American Board of Surgery Certifying Exam [11]

Lastly, practice cases early and often. Practicing cases is like practicing questions for your written tests; they are the most important aspect of your preparation. It is typically best to start doing this in your fourth year of residency and to increase your practice frequency over the course of your last 2 years. Utilize any opportunities your residency or fellowship offers for practice, whether this is in the form of organized oral board practice scenarios or just an attending coming to dedicated educational time offering to run through oral board cases. Practice cases with your co-residents or fellows or ask former residents, who just took the exam, to practice scenarios with you. In the months leading up to your CE, you should be doing practice cases daily.

Conclusion

Preparing for your general surgery examinations is a marathon, with some sprints around test time. By taking a long-term approach to these tests, anyone, regardless of their test-taking ability, can do well and succeed on these exams. Having a plan and creating positive habits are the keys to many different aspects of general surgery residency, and the ABSITE and boards are no different.

Pearls
- Take a long-term approach in preparing for the boards.
- Develop a systematic core reading plan, featuring one of the major surgical textbooks, with the goal to get through the textbook twice during a 5-year residency.
- Practice for the ABSITE and Qualifying Exam using available multiple choice study aids (e.g., SESAP®, *The ABSITE Review*, *Behind The Knife*).
- For the Certifying Exam, we recommend taking a review course.
- Review oral boards scenarios with colleagues and mentors early and often.
- Board preparation is a marathon, not a sprint.

References

1. Cameron AM. Current surgical therapy: John Cameron's contribution to surgical education and training via textbook. Ann Surg. 2018;267(2S Suppl 2):S6–9. https://doi.org/10.1097/SLA.0000000000002518.
2. Townsend C. Sabiston textbook of surgery. 21st ed. Philadelphia, PA: Elsevier; 2021. pages cm
3. Brunicardi FC, Schwartz SI. Schwartz's principles of surgery. 8th ed. New York: McGraw-Hill, Health Pub. Division; 2005. p. xv, 1950 p.
4. The Surgical Council on Resident Education Inc. https://www.surgicalcore.org/. Accessed 16 June 2022.
5. Kevin Kniery JB, McClellan J, Steele S, Kashyap M, Vu M. Behind the knife. New York: McGraw-Hill Education Medical; 2020. https://behindtheknife.org/
6. Kevin Kniery JB, McClellan J, Steele S, Kashyap M, Vu M. Behind the Knife: ABSITE podcase companion. 2nd ed. New York: Amazon Publishing; 2020.
7. Fiser SM. The ABSITE review. 7th ed. Philadelphia, PA: Wolters Kluwer; 2022. pages cm
8. Dimick JB, Upchurch GR, Sonnenday CJ. Clinical scenarios in surgery: decision making and operative technique, Clinical scenarios in surgery, vol. xxxiii. Philadelphia, PA: Wolters Kluwer Health/Lippincott Williams & Wilkins; 2012. p. 633.
9. Brad Snyder AN. How to win: on the American Board of Surgery Certifying Exam. 1st ed. Trafford Publishing; British Columbia 2009: 484.
10. Neff MA. Passing the general surgery oral board exam. 2nd ed. New York: Springer; 2013.
11. Aji S. Safe answers for the American Board of Surgery certifying exam. 5th ed. Clintwood: Safe Answers; 2000. p. 273.

Chapter 3
Talent Versus Hard Work

Devon Pace

Talent and Hard Work

Talent is a natural attribute that is defined by inherent skill. In the surgical space, this is most often exemplified by operative aptitude. In general, it is important to recognize that individuals with true operative talent are extremely rare and only represent a very small proportion of practicing surgeons. Talent must be fostered to truly see its full effect, and one nurtures this only through hard work and persistence. It is the trust and respect of the process that hone your ability in the operating room. It is focus and attention to fine detail, regardless of your level of exhaustion, that will serve you well both clinically and operatively. The surgeon must harness the ability to remain calm and collected in times of stress. Lastly, the surgeon must develop the discipline to always complete tasks the right way, no matter the consequences of time. Persistence—hard work—is what separates good surgeons from great surgeons. Truly gifted surgeons were not able to achieve their successes without this level of attentiveness.

So, how do we all get there? It starts with self-reflection and evaluation of one's own abilities to gain insight into areas that can be improved. This degree of awareness can be difficult to achieve, but practicing this skill is just as important as practicing tying with both hands. By strengthening mental awareness, one will be able to isolate key maneuvers that one can improve upon and reliably anticipate the next steps or complications that may arise during surgery. However, the surgeon in training must be confident enough to ask for direct feedback about operative skills, as it is difficult to discern these areas very early in residency. Additionally, depending on the attending surgeon, this feedback may not be provided spontaneously. Most importantly, surgeons are always learning throughout their careers and can always continue to improve.

D. Pace (✉)
Thomas Jefferson University Hospitals, Philadelphia, PA, USA

A. Ratnasekera et al. (eds.), *General Surgery Residency Survival Guide*, https://doi.org/10.1007/978-3-031-25617-2_3

Personal Accountability

It is imperative that you are your own biggest critic in and out of the operating room—to a point. Endless self-criticism without recognition of one's successes can also inhibit confidence and development. Nevertheless, it is not okay to settle for a surgical construct that "might be good enough." If you are not happy with the anastomosis, take it down and do it again. If you do not like the skin closure, cut the suture out and start over. Vince Lombardi once said, "Practice does not make perfect. Perfect practice makes perfect." Surgeons are blessed with the opportunity to make a major impact on an individual's life, and those patients have entrusted the surgeon to operate on them. It is the surgeon's duty to maintain this degree of discipline in return. This level of tenacity needs to be practiced early in residency and starts with studying for cases and simulating operative movements. These behaviors will become second nature over time, and one will see marked improvements in one's abilities with such practice.

Attitude and Modesty

These characteristics can be the most difficult to exemplify, due to fatigue, criticism, stress, and distractions. Attitude and modesty require the most mindful actions daily. Each transition through training lends the opportunity to display your abilities in a way that is admirable to the entire team, from medical students to nurses and attendings. Your approachability is what dictates how, when, and what kind of feedback you receive. You are more likely to obtain honest, direct, and constructive guidance if you remain approachable and demonstrate an ability to accept such feedback graciously. In addition, surgeons especially admire trainees that ask well-formulated questions about patient care or operative thought processes that display a deeper level of engagement. These characteristics demonstrate integrity and ownership of the respected role that surgeons possess.

The talents any given individual possesses are largely granted by providence. However, hard work, persistence, grit, and determination can likely overcome just about any deficiencies in talent. Surgeons can refine their ability to utilize self-reflection, demonstrate personal accountability, and exemplify a positive attitude. These factors make great surgeons and generally sit under the guise of "talent," but clearly these are traits that can be developed and trained.

This training process does not end at the conclusion of residency or fellowship and should be carried into one's professional career. Most importantly, have fun! Surgical residency is an extremely challenging yet also extremely rewarding opportunity and experience. Find those things that are meaningful outside of work and use those as motivators to keep going. Despite the challenge, residency is an experience that one will never forget!

Pearls
- Keep a record of cases, and log at least one thing you learned from each case.
- Ask for feedback from attendings regularly, in regard to both clinical and operative responsibilities.
- Learn to separate out the idiosyncrasies from the constructive feedback.
- Simulate the real-life scenario when practicing as best as possible (i.e., handle instruments with gloves on, tie with gloves on, tie into a coffee can).
- Focused observation leads to well-developed anticipation during cases.
- Take breaks and ask for help when you need it.
- Have fun!

Chapter 4
Acquiring Wisdom and Judgment: Good Judgment Comes from Bad Experience; Bad Experience Comes from Poor Judgment

William Preston and Sourav Podder

If there is one feature that all aspiring surgical residents have in common, it is an apprehension about being wrong. We study with our limited time off, practice our technical skills, and prepare to know everything possible about our patients. When we get it right, we are proud of the time spent in preparation. However, when we get it wrong, the predominant feelings are those of inadequacy and failure. Hence, the question eventually arises for many surgeons: "Am I cut out for this?" Many surgeons, upon reflection at the end of their residency on the personal growth they have made as doctors, argue that the most valuable lessons gained were learned in hindsight from mistakes and failures. The bridge between bad experience, in the form of failure, and good judgment is one that is imperative for surgical residents to cross, and this comes in the form of accepting that, if we let them, our failures can be our greatest teachers.

Arguably, the best quality a surgical resident can have is receptiveness to critical feedback—both from teachers and self. There are largely three drivers for medical decision-making: 1) evidence, 2) anecdotal experience, and 3) an educated guess based on the information available. Unfortunately, evidence accounts for only some of these decisions. Experience plays a large role in what we do and the decisions we make. We often learn the most from our errors. Surgeons in training (and beyond) may feel awful when these shortcomings affect patients, but conscientious surgeons learn from them and so change their practices to become more suited to treat the problem the next time it comes along.

W. Preston (✉) · S. Podder
Thomas Jefferson University Hospitals, Philadelphia, PA, USA
e-mail: William.Preston@jefferson.edu; Sourav.Podder@jefferson.edu

© The Author(s), under exclusive license to Springer Nature Switzerland AG 2023
A. Ratnasekera et al. (eds.), *General Surgery Residency Survival Guide*,
https://doi.org/10.1007/978-3-031-25617-2_4

Pearls
- After any operative case, try to take away three tangible learning points that could make you better, regardless of your level.
- Ask for feedback, after every case!
- If you make a mistake, inquire about what you did and why it was wrong, and incorporate the correct way of doing it into daily practice.
- It is okay to feel bad about an error; in fact, it probably proves that you truly care about the patient. The key is own up to it and learn from it.
- Tie at least 100 knots with each hand every day. Start off by tying to a full can of soda and work the way up to an empty one. This may seem like a lot—but challenge yourself to be better, faster, and softer with the hands.
- Be your own worst critic. Residents will experience cases where they will not get critical feedback from their attending or seniors. Residents will not be perfect— and that is okay.
- The real failure is making an error and not learning from it.

Chapter 5
Developing Surgical Skills

Madison M. Crutcher and Lisa A. Bevilacqua

Introduction

At the beginning of training, the concept of a 5-year surgical residency may feel long, but as you begin to comprehend the sheer volume and complexity of surgical diseases and operations to learn, the time in training can quickly feel inadequate. In addition to learning how to care for patients in the trauma bay, floors, and intensive care units, general surgical trainees must also learn how to operate on most areas of the human body. While increasing the number of hours available in the day is impossible, there are many ways surgical trainees can maximize the efficiency of their time in the operating room and then supplement this training on their own time. Herein are discussed the concrete steps a trainee can take to be best prepared for the OR, to optimize learning in the OR, and to reinforce learning outside of the OR.

Preoperative Preparation

1. *Use Available Resources.* Simulation and the internet have vastly expanded the ability to "practice" surgery outside the OR. Before cases, in addition to reading the steps of the operation, learners also now have access to countless video recordings of the same operations. The ability to see the anatomy prior to entering the OR as well as visual representations of the steps of the procedure are invaluable. Some tried-and-true resources include SAGES, Microsurgeon.org, and Toronto Video Atlas of Surgery.

M. M. Crutcher (✉) · L. A. Bevilacqua
Thomas Jefferson University Hospitals, Philadelphia, PA, USA

© The Author(s), under exclusive license to Springer Nature
Switzerland AG 2023
A. Ratnasekera et al. (eds.), *General Surgery Residency Survival Guide*,
https://doi.org/10.1007/978-3-031-25617-2_5

2. *Trainers.* With the growth of minimally invasive surgery, including laparoscopic, robotic, endovascular, and endoscopic approaches, the growth of available trainers has also expanded. At our home institution, we have 24/7 access to trainers for Fundamentals of Laparoscopic Surgery (FLS), Fundamentals of Endoscopic Surgery (FES), and robotics. Basic laparoscopic skills can be practiced prior to cases, increasing the chances you will be permitted to advance in the operating room. In addition, with access to the endoscopic and the robotic simulators, it is easy to familiarize yourself with how the equipment works prior to the operating room, in order not to waste time on low yield skills. Standardized curricula for FLS, FES, and robotics can be accessed at the following:

(a) FES: https://www.fesprogram.org
(b) FLS: https://www.flsprogram.org
(c) Intuitive robotic: https://www.davincisurgerycommunity.com

3. *Boot Camps.* More recently, surgical boot camps have been implemented at the medical school, residency, and fellowship levels to establish standardized preparation for trainees and allow for repeated practice of skills in a controlled, supervised environment [1].

Intraoperative

1. *Be present.* While all surgical residents would always prefer to be the one operating, it is not uncommon to be assisting in complex portions of the case. There is something to learn from all aspects of an operation. In addition, actively engaged residents are more likely to be involved by their attendings.
2. *Anticipate next steps.* Prior to arriving in the operating room, you should be familiar with the basic flow of the case. Showing that you can anticipate the next step of the case will not only improve the chances of your being allowed to progress in the operating room, but also better synthesize what you are learning. Demonstrating your knowledge can be done by asking for instruments ahead of time, providing anticipatory retraction, and asking informed questions that demonstrate your knowledge.
3. *Take Video/Film Yourself.* The majority of laparoscopic and robotic platforms are capable of recording intraoperatively. This means that you are able to record yourself performing a laparoscopic cholecystectomy, review the tape, and try to learn what you would do differently the next time. These videos can also be reviewed with an attending, who can provide additional feedback in a more secure, less stressful situation outside of the OR [2]. Keep a multi-gigabyte jump drive handy.

Postoperative

1. *Feedback.* It is important to take stock of how the case went. Either request feedback from your attending or be honest with yourself about what you did well and what you need to improve on. Several studies have evaluated the impact of feedback in the surgical setting [3].
2. *Notes.* In addition to keeping track of your personal notes from the case, write down how the case was set up and performed. The ability to review this prior to the next time you do this case will improve the flow of the operation and increase the autonomy given to you.

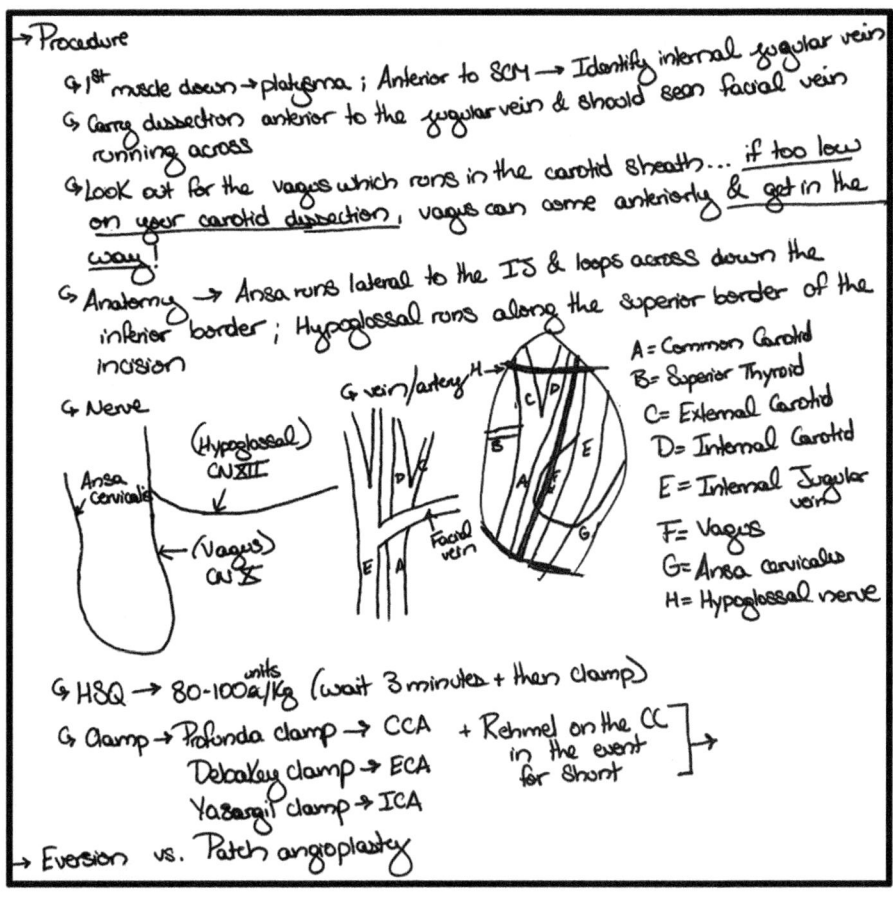

Image credit: Prashanth Palvannan, MD, MPH

3. *Repetition.* While residents may have heard the old adage "see one, do one, teach one," it is going to take more than one time doing something to become proficient. After learning a new skill before or in the OR, continue to practice it on one's own time. Do not let the only time one does a skill be on the patient. While some things are hard to simulate, even low-fidelity trainers have been shown to be effective. Simple skills like tying in a deep cavity, intracorporeal knot tying, or laparoscopic suturing can easily be practiced before or after the OR.

Conclusions

While nothing will replace the learning that takes place intraoperatively, given the increasing demands of surgical residency, it is more important than ever to come to the operating room prepared to get the most out of a case. Using the available simulators prior to the operating room, staying present and anticipating the next steps in the operating room, and continuing the practice after operating will increase the yield of each case.

Pearls
- Use available online resources (e.g., videos and descriptions of the technical steps of operations) to prepare for operative cases.
- Practice of minimally invasive surgical skills on trainers prior to your surgical cases can increase the chances that you are allowed to do more by your attending.
- Seek out or ask your residency program to create "surgical boot camps" for immersive technical training.
- Be present, and attempt to learn from every part of the case, even if you are not the one performing the steps.
- Seek feedback directly after each case.
- Record video of your operations for later review, and take notes and diagrams (particularly of more complex cases).

References

1. Bevilacqua LA, Simon J, Rutigliano D, Sorrento J, Wackett A, Chandran L, et al. Surgical boot camp for fourth-year medical students: impact on objective skills and subjective confidence. Surgery. 2020;167(2):298–301.
2. Dedhia PH, Barrett M, Ives G, Magas CP, Varban OA, Wong SL, et al. Intraoperative feedback: a video-based analysis of faculty and resident perceptions. J Surg Educ. 2019;76(4):906–15.
3. El Boghdady M, Alijani A. Feedback in surgical education. Surgeon. 2017;15(2):98–103.

Chapter 6
Effective Methods and Tools for Studying

Darshak Thosani and Micaela Collins

Introduction

During general surgery residency, studying does not take the form one may be accustomed to after college and medical school. It will not involve weeks or even days of dedicated study time. Instead, one must recognize the learning opportunities every day at work and spend time outside work reinforcing and expanding on what has already been learned. Studying while balancing a challenging residency schedule involves developing a routine and making a conscious effort to study something relevant daily. Despite how daunting this task may seem, there are a few resources and methods of studying that are helpful for both general surgical knowledge and conquering the yearly American Board of Surgery In-Training Examination (ABSITE).

Variety of Resources

The most important part of studying effectively during residency is finding the resources that work best for each particular resident. As seen in Table 6.1, there are multiple options for textbooks, question banks, and resources for learning operative techniques—and this list is not all-inclusive. A question bank or textbook in isolation is insufficient. To be successful, one must draw from multiple categories of resources.

D. Thosani (✉) · M. Collins
Thomas Jefferson University Hospitals, Philadelphia, PA, USA
e-mail: darshak.thosani@jefferson.edu; Micaela.collins@jefferson.edu

© The Author(s), under exclusive license to Springer Nature
Switzerland AG 2023
A. Ratnasekera et al. (eds.), *General Surgery Residency Survival Guide*,
https://doi.org/10.1007/978-3-031-25617-2_6

Table 6.1 Studying resources

Reading resources
Cameron's Current Surgical Therapy
Sabiston Textbook of Surgery
Schwartz Principles of Surgery
Mulholland & Greenfield's Surgery: Scientific Principles and Practice
The ABSITE Review by Fiser*
Behind The Knife ABSITE Podcasts and Review Book*
The Surgical Review: An Integrated Basic and Clinical Science Study Guide*
(*Denotes ABSITE Review Book)
Question banks
ABSITE Quest
SCORE (Surgical Council on Resident Education)
TrueLearn ABSITE
Learn operative techniques
Operative Dictations in General and Vascular Surgery
Fischer's Mastery of Surgery
YouTube or other source of operative videos online

It should be a goal to finish at least one general surgery textbook over the course of residency. Some of the more popular texts are Cameron's, Sabiston's, Schwartz's, and Greenfield's. Each varies in the level of detail and the way in which the content is delivered, but any of them will suffice. The most important part is picking the textbook that one finds easy to read and comprehend. Amazon offers a preview option for each of these textbooks, and spending a few minutes reading each book will give one a better understanding of which resource might be most suitable to purchase.

Aside from a major textbook, it is helpful to use a review book for the ABSITE. Three options that each provide an excellent synopsis of heavily covered ABSITE topics are Fiser's, Behind The Knife, and The Surgical Review. Fiser's and The Surgical Review focus on basic science and physiology, with the latter being more detailed. Behind The Knife is more clinically focused and offers accompanying podcasts created by fellow general surgery residents who have mastered the yearly ABSITE.

Question banks are arguably the most important resource if only for their flexibility: one can fit in a few questions anytime or anywhere on a mobile phone, tablet, or computer. It is of paramount importance to read the explanations provided for each question, even when one answers the question correctly. Without this, question banks are a wasted resource. Three of the question banks recommended are ABSITE Quest (AQ), TrueLearn, and SCORE. AQ is unique in that it delivers five questions daily to one's phone. Residents using AQ are able to keep on track with studying without being overburdened. AQ's drawback is that a resident cannot do more than five questions in 1 day.

TrueLearn and SCORE are more traditional question banks that are self-paced and allow the user to select how many questions to do at a given time. TrueLearn provides longer explanations to each question as well as links to outside resources.

The answer explanations in SCORE are shorter, but each topic is accompanied by modules written by experts in the field. None of the three question banks are the perfect resource, but they all provide questions relating to every topic covered on the yearly ABSITE. Your choice may be swayed by what your residency program provides for free. Regardless of the question bank, doing questions will cement the understanding of topics and make learning a little every day convenient.

Finally, studying surgery requires preparation for every surgical case. It is important to know the steps, anatomy, and potential complications for surgeries to be effective and safe in the operating room (OR). If you can demonstrate knowledge and understanding of the steps to a procedure, attendings will be more likely to grant increased autonomy in the OR. It can be useful to use the Internet to find videos of the surgery you will be performing. Additionally, Operative Dictations and Fischer's textbook provide the steps of most major cases along with pictures in the case of the latter.

Methods of Studying

By the start of surgical residency, most individuals have an idea of what type of learners they are. For example, one may learn best by doing questions or by listening to lectures/podcasts. Knowing this will allow one to focus attention on the resources that are most effective. Regardless, it is best to study daily. Whether that is 15 minutes or 2 hours, the consistency of learning or reviewing something every day will be beneficial for retaining and utilizing the knowledge. In addition, it is easy to be overwhelmed by the breadth of general surgery and the number of available resources. Spending a few minutes each day on a given topic or just a handful of questions helps break down the daunting field of general surgery into smaller, more manageable pieces. Develop a routine, but be sure not to overestimate the amount of time available for studying after a day at work. Finally, understand that one will not always be able to stick to a proposed schedule because of a late operative case or consult at work. Do not be discouraged by a missed day or two—pick up where one left off, and with diligence, one will be able to cover what is necessary in the long run.

When it comes to questions, it is recommended doing 5–20 questions daily. As interns, doing 5 questions daily will likely be enough, as many questions will involve new topics to an intern. Interns should not expect to ace the practice questions, but will notice that as they advance through residency, they will recognize more topics and score better. Given that, as one progresses through residency, one should be able to answer questions faster and be able to do more than 5 questions a day.

Aside from questions, it is recommended that residents read a portion of a textbook chapter or review a topic encountered at work daily. Doing this will reinforce clinical experiences and provide a greater context for what has been encountered at work. Spacing out learning by committing to tackling only a little bit every day is the most effective technique for retaining knowledge and finding the time to study with a tiring residency schedule.

Along with developing a studying routine, it is equally important to make time to devote to self-care, whether that is exercising, spending time with friends or family, dining out, or whatever hobbies make you happiest. Some days, you will have to forego studying to prioritize these activities, but balance is key to avoid getting burnt out. Finally, whenever possible, try to maintain good sleep hygiene and get the sleep you need to function. Overall, general surgery residency involves long hours, a plethora of knowledge to be learned, and very little free time. Nevertheless, these resources and advice can provide you with the tools to succeed in any residency program.

Pearls
- Do 5–20 questions every day, and do NOT get discouraged if you are not getting them correct.
- Question banks should be viewed as a learning tool, not a test of knowledge. Again, for them to be a useful resource, you must read the explanations.
- Endeavor to find a textbook early in residency that you find easy to digest and comprehend.
- Everyone studies at a different pace and with different methods. You should NOT get discouraged if a colleague is doing "more."
- Focus on learning while on the job and using study resources to consolidate and expand on what is encountered clinically.
- Do not view studying as a burden, but rather as a tool to become a better diagnostician and surgeon for patients.
- There may be days when self-care (in whatever form you prefer) is a better use of limited time than studying. Residency can be grueling—learn to recognize when you need time off to avoid burnout and fatigue.

Chapter 7
Research

Ryan Lamm

Types of Research

Each of us would love to be the lead scientist that discovers the "cure" for cancer or designs a randomized control trial to prove once and for all which mesh is the "best" for hernia repair. Unfortunately, the challenge (and number one resource in medical school and residency) is *time*. In an already packed schedule, one needs to choose the project that one has enough time to complete. This means nights, weekends, and in between cases when necessary. Hand in hand comes the notion that these projects need to be something that one is passionate about as well, or one will undoubtedly push the project to the side and it will never be completed. At the end of the day, an incomplete project is equivalent to never having done the project in the eyes of application reviewers and job interviewers. How do we know which type of project is best for us? Figure 7.1 lists the most common types of research in the general surgery realm and places them on a spectrum of time and academic yield.

As the graph shows, projects which involve basic science and randomized control trials (RCTs) can take on the order of years, but can yield high academic impact. On the other end of the spectrum, case reports/case series take less time (days to weeks), but yield lower impact. While this graph is not all-encompassing, medical students and residents should choose projects that are feasible for them to complete in the time they have available. Importantly, it is also an option to join a team/project that has already begun work or will continue after one's training period is complete. Projects involving national datasets (i.e., National Inpatient Sample (NIS), National Surgical Quality Improvement Program (NSQIP), as well as many others) are most common because with the right team, one can take the least amount of time

R. Lamm (✉)
Thomas Jefferson University Hospitals, Philadelphia, PA, USA

© The Author(s), under exclusive license to Springer Nature Switzerland AG 2023
A. Ratnasekera et al. (eds.), *General Surgery Residency Survival Guide*,
https://doi.org/10.1007/978-3-031-25617-2_7

Fig. 7.1 Types of research
by time and academic yield

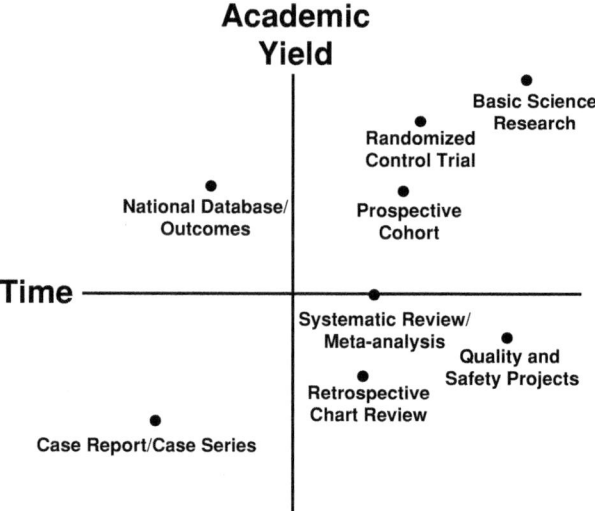

and produce the highest academic yield due to large sample sizes available [1]. Choosing the correct database is a team effort, and taking the time to research the scope, variables available, and previous work performed is well worth it.

Roles of a Research Team

Assembling a research team is vital for success. Below is a basic list of roles necessary to complete a successful project:

(a) *Principal Investigator (PI)*: This role is generally filled by an attending physician, in charge of design and decision-making, and who will be the last/senior author on any publication/presentation.

(b) *Coordinator*: This role is in charge of organizing the project and data and oftentimes coordinating when the team will meet to progress the project.

(c) *Statistician*: Most projects (except case report/series) will involve some form of statistics; various members will have different levels of training, but it is important to designate who will be in charge of data analysis and what level of analysis will be required; a fatal flaw is not having someone who can perform the level of statistics required.

(d) *Primary Author*: This is the role most commonly filled by the medical student or resident; this role requires involvement in project design and being the contact person for any issues and head writer of abstracts, posters, presentations, and manuscripts.

(e) *Secondary Authors and Team Members*: This is the second most commonly filled role by medical students or residents, who aid the primary author in all roles mentioned above; this role is more appropriate if less time is available.

Of note, one person can fill two or more of these roles, but a project without these roles will almost certainly fail (or will be very painful to complete). Time and effort requirements will vary depending on the type of research project being performed.

Manuscript Writing

So, when all the data is collected, the statistician has provided the p values. Now what? Nothing is more daunting than the blinking cursor on an empty page waiting for one to fill it with the fruit of one's hard work. Luckily, the elements of a strong (and, thus, accepted) manuscript are the same: abstract, introduction, methods and materials, results, discussion, and conclusion. While there are many resources that attempt to simplify the process, one extremely succinct and useful one is a chapter by Ibrahim and Dimick on writing for impact [2]. It is worthwhile to read in its entirety, but the main message is to stick to a high-yield formula in each section and chip away at what one can, when one has time and energy. Sometimes, this means writing results first to drive the narrative of the introduction and discussion; sometimes, this means writing the methods first, since at the point of writing, these will not change. The important thing is to start writing! Remember that when writing a draft of a manuscript, it is just that—a DRAFT. Many rounds of editing will create the polished product we are used to reading in journals, and the sooner one completes each section, the sooner one can get it out to team members to review, edit, and eventually submit.

Publishing

One made it through the manuscript drafting phase and is ready to select a platform to submit a project. Hooray! Again, now what? Publishing comes in the form of abstracts to conferences, which can lead to poster or oral presentations at local or national conferences and manuscripts in peer-reviewed journals. Principal investigators are a great resource to determine deadlines for local and national conferences, which can help you share one's work in the field and add to one's CV. They can also help determine which journal is the best "fit" for one's project. Referring to Fig. 7.1 again, certain journals are only looking for certain types of study on this graph. Another important concept to understand is a journal's impact factor—which is a numeric score of the average number of times an article printed in the journal is cited in a year—which can guide residents to submit their projects to an appropriate journal [3]. Finally, do not get discouraged if one's first attempt to publish is rejected! A recent study found that greater than 60% of published articles were rejected by one or more journals prior to the one that agreed to publish [4]. Take the reviewer's feedback, consult with the team, and put one's hard work out there again!

While this chapter has been a whirlwind overview of research as a medical student or resident, the takeaways include choosing the right project, team, and strategy to take a project from a great idea to a published manuscript. Most importantly, choose something one is passionate about; this will help bring the project over the finish line. Below are some pearls from this chapter to remember.

Pearls
- Time = most valuable resource.
- Incomplete project = no project.
- National database/outcome research is most common because it takes the "least" amount of time and yields the highest academic impact.
- Choosing the correct database is a team effort, and taking the time to research the scope, variables available, and previous work performed is well worth it.
- Successful projects have personnel to fill the principal investigator, coordinator, statistician, and primary author roles at a minimum.
- When writing a draft of manuscript, remember that it is just that, a DRAFT; many rounds of editing will polish and trim the paper to a finalized product.
- Principal investigators are a great resource to determine deadlines for local/national conferences, which can help share one's work in the field and add to one's CV.
- Do not get discouraged if the manuscript gets rejected! 60% of published articles were rejected by one or more journals prior to the one that agreed to publish.

References

1. Alluri RK, Leland H, Heckmann N. Surgical research using national databases. Ann Transl Med. 2016;4(20):393.
2. Ibrahim AM, Dimick JB. Writing for impact: how to prepare a journal article. Medical and Scientific Publishing: Elsevier; 2018. p. 81–92.
3. McKiernan EC, Schimanski LA, Nieves CM, Matthias L, Niles MT, Alperin JP. Meta-research: use of the journal impact factor in academic review, promotion, and tenure evaluations. elife. 2019;8:e47338.
4. Khadilkar SS. Rejection blues: why do research papers get rejected? J Obstet Gynaecol India. 2018;68(4):239–41.

Chapter 8
Curriculum Vitae Preparation

Uzma Rahman

Introduction

A *curriculum vitae*, or CV, is in many cases the first impression that an employer or institution has of a prospective employee or trainee. It is an important document that showcases the resident's professional achievements, skills, and experiences [1]. Therefore, developing a quality CV is an integral step towards making professional connections and propelling one's career in the right direction. CVs usually consist of multiple pages to include the resident's professional journey during residency, medical school, and other important accomplishments in the past. In contrast, a resume is more succinct, usually a page, highlighting the aspects most relevant to the position that one is applying for. A good CV can be a gateway to success. Herein is discussed when, what, and how to build a quality CV.

When to work on your CV?

- NOW! If you only had a resume in the past, start working towards a CV now. Identify the areas on the CV that need more development and start working towards filling these gaps. For example, if you do not have adequate research experience, seek opportunities to engage in research early.
- Revisit and update the CV at least every 6 months.
- Go over the CV annually with a mentor, and identify ways to make it more impactful for the following year.
- A CV that has been refined gradually and thoughtfully over time is likely to be more impactful than one that was put together overnight.

U. Rahman (✉)
Thomas Jefferson University Hospitals, Philadelphia, PA, USA
e-mail: Uzma.Rahman@jefferson.edu

© The Author(s), under exclusive license to Springer Nature Switzerland AG 2023
A. Ratnasekera et al. (eds.), *General Surgery Residency Survival Guide*,
https://doi.org/10.1007/978-3-031-25617-2_8

What to include in your CV?

- Although it is acceptable for a CV to be 2–3 pages, avoid listing irrelevant or trivial activities to fill the space.
- Throughout training, one should build meaningful accomplishments and experiences worthy of including in the CV.
- Personal information: A CV usually starts with personal information, such as full name, professional e-mail, and phone number. Including address is optional—it can be favorable if it shows ties to the location of training or employment for which one is applying.
- Education: List the most recent educational qualification first (residency training in this case), followed by medical school, any other graduate training, and finally undergraduate training. Mention the degree earned, dates attended, and location for each of these places of education. Awards and honors earned during this time can be mentioned in a separate category if multiple or included in the education section.
- Professional work: This includes previous employment or extracurricular involvements that either are relevant to the position one is applying for or demonstrate important skills, for example, committee memberships, organizing teaching sessions for medical students, volunteering at a refugee center, or running a business.
- Research: List all publications, presentations (oral and poster), abstracts, and grants here. Publications that are accepted but not yet published should be mentioned as "in press" [2]. One can arrange this section chronologically or based on the order of authorship. Grants should be listed in the final section. Grant information should include the name of the principal investigator, individual's role or percent contribution to the project, awarding institution, amount, project name, and duration of the grant.
- Academic societies and certifications: List professional memberships and any certifications you earned during training.
- Professional references: These may be listed at the end of the CV [1, 2]. Usually, two or three professional references should be listed, including people with whom one has worked closely and can attest to one's professionalism, work ethics, and caliber. For residents, one of these must be the residency program director [1]. Most importantly, notify and obtain permission from these references so that they agree to be listed as such.
- Hobbies and interests are optional to include in the CV.

How to build and refine your CV?

- When applicable, research the target role, position, or institution before constructing the CV. Pay attention to the skills and experience that the recruiter is looking for and construct the CV such that your experiences demonstrate that you are a great fit for their team.
- It is not just what information the CV contains but also how one presents this information. Keep the CV organized and use consistent chronology through different sections [2]. It should be easy to read and follow, without any unnecessary embellishments such as different fonts or colors.

- Follow the institutional guidelines, if available, to modify the CV for that specific position or institution for which one is applying [3].
- Use the same font throughout the entire CV with the size of the font varying with the section. For example, using 18 point for name, 12–14 point for headings, and 10–12 point for contents within each heading is generally acceptable. Keep it simple with standard black text against a white background.
- Proofread to eliminate any grammatical, spelling, or punctuation errors. An avoidable typing error, although seemingly insignificant, can be seen as lack of attention to detail.
- Get feedback on your CV from a trusted peer or mentor.
- You should always have a CV ready to be submitted. However, when time permits, focus on activities that are more relevant and specific for the position for which you are applying.
- A well-written cover letter, although not mandatory, is a powerful tool to support the CV. You can use it tactfully to advocate for yourself, justify or fill gaps in the CV, tie your experiences to the job position you are interested in, or provide an opportunity to the reader to learn more about you.

Conclusion

A CV narrates the applicant's professional story, accomplishments, and experiences. It represents the applicant before potential employers and professional colleagues. Therefore, it is an important document that should be curated thoughtfully and evolved over time.

Pearls
- Start working on a CV early in your career even if it is not well developed yet.
- Identify the areas on the CV that need more development and engage in professional activities that fill these voids.
- Update the CV about every 6 months.
- Remember that a good CV is curated thoughtfully over time.
- Invest time in writing a cover letter when applicable.

References

1. Agha R, Whitehurst K, Jafree D, Devabalan Y, Koshy K, Gundogan B. How to write a medical CV. Int J Surg Oncol (NY). 2017;2(6):e32. https://doi.org/10.1097/IJ9.0000000000000032.
2. Waseem M, Schnapp BH. Preparing a curriculum vitae for new graduates. AEM Educ Train. 2019;4(Suppl 1):S143–6. https://doi.org/10.1002/aet2.10420.
3. Jericho BG, Ilgen JS, Gottlieb-Smith R, Simpson D, Sullivan GM. How to write your curriculum vitae. J Grad Med Educ. 2019;11(3):333–4. https://doi.org/10.4300/JGME-D-19-00221.1.

Chapter 9
Tools for Purchase to Succeed in Residency

Lindsay Weil

Introduction

Studying and practicing skills are a critical part of general surgery residency. However, since there is little free time left in the day to dedicate to studying, it is important to find resources that allow for quick, directed, and efficient learning and practice. Below is information about tools residents find most useful for daily success during residency (Table 9.1). While this chapter focuses on many resources, it is not all-inclusive.

Table 9.1 Summary of tools for purchase

Resource	Where to find it	Current pricing
ABSITE Quest	Website: https://absitequest.com/ App: Download from a smartphone's app store	Standard package: $149 per academic year Plus package: $199 per academic year Premium package: $299 per academic year
Anki	Website: https://ankiweb.net/ App: Download from a smartphone's app store	Website: Free Android phone app: Free IOS phone app: $25 for a lifetime use
Behind The Knife	Website: https://behindtheknife.org/ Podcast: Stream from any audio streaming service	Podcast: Free ABSITE Companion book: $49.99

(continued)

L. Weil (✉)
Thomas Jefferson University Hospitals, Philadelphia, PA, USA

© The Author(s), under exclusive license to Springer Nature Switzerland AG 2023
A. Ratnasekera et al. (eds.), *General Surgery Residency Survival Guide*,
https://doi.org/10.1007/978-3-031-25617-2_9

Table 9.1 (continued)

Resource	Where to find it	Current pricing
Clinical Scenarios in Surgery	Available anywhere books are sold	New hardcopy: $145 on Amazon
Loupes	Contact residency program coordinator to be put in contact with the sales representative from desired company	Range based on company and specific products but usually around $800–$1000
Score	Website: https://www.surgicalcore.org/ App: Download from a smartphone's app store	Free with log-in from residency program
TrueLearn	Website: https://truelearn.com/general-surgery/absite-exam/ App: Download from a smartphone's app store	$369 for a 1-year ABSITE SmartBank subscription $419 for a 1-year ABSITE SmartBank + Predictive Assessment Exam
SESAP®	Website: https://www.facs.org/for-medical-professionals/education/tools-and-platforms/sesap-17/	$357 for the question bank. Best bought during fourth and fifth years of residency

ABSITE Quest

ABSITE Quest is one of the best resources available that allows for efficient study that will improve a resident's basic clinical knowledge and prepare residents for the ABSITE exam. Every day, the application delivers five high-yield ABSITE review questions directly to the subscriber's smartphone. Each question has detailed and well-referenced answers and will continue to appear until a specific topic is mastered. Due to the repetitive and condensed nature of the app, ABSITE Quest helps residents establish a productive study routine, even with a busy schedule.

ABSITE Quest is available for purchase online and is available in app form, allowing for easy access studying on a smartphone. The standard, most recommended package currently costs $149 per academic year and includes access to the full question bank as well as performance insights. It also includes a complementary increase in daily ABSITE questions as the exam nears. Other packages include a mock ABSITE exam and a 2-day comprehensive ABSITE review course that can be purchased for an additional cost.

Anki

Anki is both a website and phone application that allows residents to make intelligent flash cards custom-made to unique learning styles. Anki allows full control of the card content, layout, and review timing. Similar to ABSITE Quest, if a resident continually gets the same question wrong, it will appear more frequently. When a card or subject is mastered, it will appear less frequently. It is recommended to download on a smartphone because it allows for easy access studying during moments of downtime throughout a shift as well as at home. The Anki website and the Android app are free, while the IOS version currently costs $25 for a life-time use.

Behind The Knife

Behind The Knife (BTK) is a comprehensive surgery education podcast designed for healthcare providers at all stages of their training and career. It focuses on a wide range of surgery topics, from conversations with experts in surgical subspecialties to journal discussions and board reviews. There are even episodes dedicated to intern survival tips. One of the most useful aspects of BTK is their annual ABSITE review podcasts. The podcasts are dedicated to each system and focus on high yield facts and quick hits to increase scores and enhance learning.

Many residents utilize their time wisely by listening to the podcast on their work commute. While the podcast itself is free, it is recommended that visual learners purchase the Behind The Knife ABSITE Podcast Companion book currently being sold for $49.99. For high-level study, senior residents should also look to purchase BTK's General Surgery and Vascular Surgery Oral Board reviews.

Clinical Scenarios in Surgery

Part of being a successful resident involves having a consistent reading plan through-out the year. There are many textbooks that residents find helpful, and much of picking the right textbook is based on individual learning styles. Clinical Scenarios in Surgery is unique because it is written in a case-based approach, which appeals to many residents.

Each chapter starts with a patient presentation and then works its way through the differential diagnosis, workup, diagnosis and treatment, preoperative care, sur-gical approach, and postoperative management. While describing the surgical approach, this book provides visuals and discusses the fundamental steps to the operation, potential pitfalls, and special intraoperative considerations. While it is great for board exam preparation, these specifics allow residents to use this resource to prepare daily for the operating room and increase critical thinking skills that are required of all general surgeons. This book can be bought anywhere books are sold. It currently costs $145 for a new hardback copy on Amazon. There are also used and Kindle versions available for purchase.

Loupes

Many residents find buying loupes during their second or third year helpful. While not a necessity, loupes improve clarity, focus, and visibility during challenging cases. Loupes often allow more confidence with intraoperative skills, which can lead to more trust and autonomy in the operating room.

Loupes can be purchased through many different companies, and sometimes hospitals have a deal with one in particular. Some of the most common and reputable are Designs for Vision, SurgiTel, and Orascoptic (formerly known as Surgical Acuity). While loupes are around $1000, residency programs typically provide an education stipend which can be used toward this purchase.

Question Banks

In medical school, UWorld is heavily used for exam preparation; however, it does not have a general surgery-specific question bank. There are other tools that are more reliable for this stage of study. Each resource provides unique positives and negatives for general surgery residents.

- SCORE is an online resource that provides residents with a structured curriculum for self-learning. SCORE has its own online modules as well as a question bank. The benefit of SCORE is that the content is the most similar to ABSITE. Another benefit of SCORE is that it is typically offered for free through residency programs. Keep in mind that, unlike other resources, this question bank does not always provide thorough explanations.
- TrueLearn is another resource that residents find helpful in supplementing their studying. It includes detailed and well-referenced explanations and is the most similarly structured question bank to UWorld. Additionally, TrueLearn gives analytics regarding an individual's overall performance compared to residents across the country. Notably, the questions are typically more detailed than the content found on ABSITE. The standard package currently costs $369 for a 1-year subscription. Thirty-day, 90-day, and 180-day subscriptions are offered as well, which may align better with individual study schedules.

The Surgical Education and Self-Assessment Program (SESAP®) offered by the American College of Surgeons is considered the most similar to the Qualifying Exam. Most residents save this question bank for their fourth and fifth years of residency to use during dedicated QE studying. The standard package currently costs $357 for the full question bank.

Pearls
- ABSITE Quest is one of the best tools available for efficient study and preparation for the ABSITE and Qualifying Exam.
- Anki, Behind The Knife, and Clinical Scenarios are also valuable learning and test preparation tools.
- Consider purchasing loupes during the second or third surgical residency year; most residencies have a stipend available to help cover the cost for these devices.
- Question banks such as UWorld, SCORE, TrueLearn, and SESAP® have different advantages and disadvantages; each may be valuable but should be evaluated before purchase to ensure that the bank's format suits one's style of study/learning.

Part II
Clinical Duties

Chapter 10
Office Hours

Madison Harris

Office hours provide a window into each specialty outside of the operating room. Time in the office gives us the opportunity to see the "lifestyle" and workflow of each field. If you are prepared and engaged, office hours can be equally as rewarding as operating.

Office hours do not have to be the dreaded part of the week. Rather, they are an integral part of residency that can guide you toward your future specialty choice. Time in the office gives residents the opportunity to see the so-called lifestyle of each specialty. They can help you determine the type of patients you want to work with and the diagnoses you may want to treat. It also gives you an idea of the workflow of how these patients are seen, managed, and processed. Perhaps you want to deal with cancer diagnoses, or want to prioritize counseling patients, or will find a passion in performing office procedures. Just like evaluating hospitals for your residency program, evaluate office hours of each specialty when considering your career choices.

There are a few things to gauge when preparing for office hours. First, and foremost, find out what time they start and be on time (get there early). Try to get a copy of the patient list the day before. Familiarize yourself with the diagnoses you might come across and treatment options to impress your attending. Along with the schedule of the day, it is also important to consider the nuances such as what to wear: business casual vs. scrubs, whether a white coat is necessary, and whether you will get a lunch break if it is a full day of patients. It may seem trivial but walking into an office in scrubs while everyone else is in slacks is not a confidence booster. Pro tip: keep an extra granola bar in your pocket and a spare white coat in your locker/car.

M. Harris (✉)
Christiana Care Health System, Newark, DE, USA
e-mail: madison.harris@christianacare.org

A. Ratnasekera et al. (eds.), *General Surgery Residency Survival Guide*,
https://doi.org/10.1007/978-3-031-25617-2_10

Office hours are a unique window into understanding how patients are seen, evaluated, referred to, and counseled for surgery. Be engaged and spend time talking with patients. Understand their background, what type of work up is needed, what referrals are needed to be performed prior to scheduling surgery or other interventions, what type of follow-up they need after having surgery and after leaving the hospital, and what type of preventative screening practices are necessary for a particular patient population. Learning all these aspects is vital to our surgical education. With a busy surgical schedule, we can often palpate the ticking clock during our inpatient conversations. Office hours are the time to perfect your deliverance of information and to learn treatment plans for a myriad of diagnoses. When discussing surgical options, it is a wonderful time to hone in on communication of risks and benefits, which is something we as residents may not get the opportunity to do in detail in a more chaotic acute inpatient setting. It is also a fun time to stir up conversations with attendings outside of the operating room. Do not be afraid to ask questions and learn about the routine of the specialty. Who knows, maybe you will score a coffee and riveting conversation from your attending when the day is done!

Pearls
- Office hours can give you insight to a specialty and may guide you toward your future career.
- Be prepared.
- Do not be afraid to ask questions.

Chapter 11
Triaging Clinical Duties and Being Organized

Benjamin A. Dixson and Brone S. Lobichusky

Introduction

A significant portion of your success early on in general surgery residency is based on your ability to demonstrate organizing and triaging clinical duties. This chapter discusses key concepts to promote growth in these areas.

Anticipation

A smooth day or night starts at sign-out, arguably the most important time of the day, with the handoff of important patient care information. When chart reviewing, anticipate which patients may worsen clinically or require interventions. In the beginning, it will be helpful to ask the outgoing team or chief which patients they are concerned may develop complications and a general game plan including anticipatory guidance from the team that knows that patient best. This includes everything from urinary retention after Foley removal to postoperative tachycardia. As issues arise, it will then be easier to triage them and conduct a workup. An important part to an efficient and accurate sign-out is making sure whatever handoff tool (i.e., patient list) your residency program uses is as up to date and accurate as possible prior to starting the sign-out process so the incoming team does not have inaccurate information to cloud their clinical decisions.

B. A. Dixson (✉)
ChristianaCare Health System, Newark, DE, USA
e-mail: benjamin.dixson@christianacare.org

B. S. Lobichusky
WellSpan Health, York, PA, USA
e-mail: blobichusky@wellspan.org

Least to Most Stable

Use the trauma "ABCs" and hemodynamic stability to determine which patients should be seen first. Any patient with a new oxygen requirement (airway), shortness of breath (breathing), incisional bleeding, tachycardia/bradycardia, or hypotension (circulation) *must* be a priority for you to respond to the patient's bedside for rapid evaluation. If you are unable to see a patient immediately, order the workup—imaging and/or labs—when you receive the page. This can buy time and enable you to have all the supplemental information when you are able to evaluate the patient. Certain EMRs enable alerts to be set when results are completed, or you can ask the nurses to page you.

A key skill to develop is an overall understanding of the urgency of a task. Not every page you get as an intern will be equal. Apart from unstable patients (ABCs), there will be varying degrees of urgency to the tasks you have in a given day. Here are some principles that can help you triage these tasks appropriately:

- Highest urgency: Decompensating patients with abnormalities in their ABCs. For example: Coding patient.
- High urgency: Tasks that will directly affect patient care within the next hour. For example: Communicating to nursing staff the timing of stopping a patient's heparin drip prior to a semi-urgent surgery to prevent intraoperative and postoperative bleeding.
- High urgency: Consults in the emergency department (ED), unless you are tied up with an unstable patient, help streamline patient care. Of course, unstable consults should be seen as soon as possible, but even low-acuity patients in the ED should be seen as soon as you are able.
- Moderate urgency: If a nurse pages you repeatedly with concerns about an otherwise stable patient, it is best to go to the bedside to evaluate the patient and address the nurse's concerns. Sometimes, there is a legitimate problem with the patient or there is a misunderstanding that can be clarified to reassure the patient and/or nurse.
- Low urgency: Ordering routine labs for the following day, as this can be done at any time up to about 30 min before you want the labs to be drawn.

Bundle Tasks

Some of the most time-consuming tasks are order updates. Whether pharmacy is paging to change antibiotic dosing or nurses are asking to renew telemetry, these nonurgent but important tasks can easily accumulate. There are two ways to tackle such pages.

- Address them readily as they come in. They can be quick tasks and are a satisfying check mark on your to-do list. However, it is very easy to become glued to a computer opening multiple charts and editing various order sets. It may also not be feasible to expeditiously access a computer when in the trauma bay or placing an NG tube.

- Save these tasks for when you have a brief free period. Sitting down at a computer can provide a nice reprieve and is an excellent time to chart review. *Answer all pages as they come in.* It is courteous and will benefit you to let the nurse know that you are currently occupied but understand the issue and will get to it within the next 30 min. The person on the other end of the phone is generally understanding but can also stress if it is an urgent concern which they feel should be addressed more immediately. When your more life-threatening issues are addressed, you can check off the boxes for the more minor tasks all at one time.
- If you are out on the wards completing tasks of relatively equal urgency, it is wise to develop an organized path (such as starting on the highest floor and working down to the lowest floor or vice versa) to be efficient rather than unnecessarily running all over the hospital and backtracking several times.

Communicate

All senior residents appreciate early, ongoing, and honest communication. If you have the slightest bit of uncertainty regarding the acuity of a patient issue or how to begin a workup, let one of your seniors know immediately. They will be able to guide you in next steps, plus this will alert them to a potential emergency. It never hurts to "load the boat." The same ongoing communication is important with nurses. If you are talking with a nurse from the surgical floor, it will behoove you to ask him or her if other nurses have messages for you. Not only will this save you time from returning multiple separate pages, but it will also save the nurses from tracking you down and can make patient care, overall, more efficient.

Pearls
- General surgery residency is a season of training where you will often have multiple pending duties, and part of your educational experience is to grow to learn how to triage these duties appropriately.
- Organization keeps you focused on the tasks that need to be accomplished before the day ends and gives you the framework to ensure that things do not slip through the cracks.
- Do your best to completely finish tasks prior to moving on to the next task, when able.

Chapter 12
Surviving Call

Zi L. Huang

The sun has set, and your colleagues have retreated home. Four members, including yourself, stayed behind to keep the fire alive. The chief resident and attending surgeon are sweating in the operating room (OR) #6 attempting to control a duodenal hemorrhage refractory to endoscopic intervention and embolization by interventional radiology; tensions are high, and massive transfusion protocol is activated. The intensive care unit surgery resident is actively resuscitating bed #2, multisystemic trauma with an open abdomen that suddenly coded.

You just triaged three emergency department (ED) stat consults, deciding to prioritize an elderly female presenting in septic shock with imaging demonstrating obvious pneumoperitoneum. Running down the northeast stairwell, you scroll through electronic medical records on your phone to review the patient's surgical/medical history. Suddenly, your hospital phone buzzes. The floor intern is frantically describing a bariatric patient who is postoperative day #3 from her bypass, acutely tachycardic to 140, and febrile to 102 and complains of chest pain.

As you explain the most appropriate labs and imaging modality, the ED hallway screens flash red/black. Trauma alert is activated, and your pager once again screams for your attention. *GUN SHOT WOUNDS, TRAUMA UNKNOWN, INTUBATED, 5 MINUTES.* You silently shout profanity down a hallway cluttered by empty beds, carts, and mobile X-ray devices and force yourself to take a deep breath. You remembered that you were not alone.

You call the operating room front desk to deliver an SOS message to OR #6 and sprint to the trauma bay. At least 13 other healthcare colleagues are looking to you for instructions. You have done this before, and this is only another Tuesday night. You identify yourself and initiate crew resource management to prepare for the worst-case scenario.

Z. L. Huang (✉)
WellSpan Health, York, PA, USA
e-mail: zhuang@wellspan.org

© The Author(s), under exclusive license to Springer Nature
Switzerland AG 2023
A. Ratnasekera et al. (eds.), *General Surgery Residency Survival Guide*,
https://doi.org/10.1007/978-3-031-25617-2_12

General surgery call is inherently chaotic; our job is to embrace and organize the chaos. Here are the practical tips that will help you become an effective general surgery resident.

Utilize the EMR: The hospital electronic health/medical record system has the function of creating and managing a private list of patients. Document and keep a clear list, electronic if possible, so it is not lost in the chaos. This list should include new consults, patients with worsening clinical status, and patients with pending tasks. Actively review this list throughout the night to follow up and progress patient care. This list will also serve as your sign-out list to respective colleagues in the morning.

Triage every new patient brought to your attention. You will learn and hone this skill with endless hours in the hospital. Always prioritize the sickest patient first. This obvious fact often eludes the junior residents during real-life applications because not all tasks are created equal. Patient care comes before nonurgent documentation. If documentation is required to facilitate operative intervention, it is acceptable to abbreviate. Assessment/plan may say nothing more than "Patient presented in septic shock with pneumoperitoneum of unknown origin. Ongoing resuscitation. Broad-spectrum antibiotics. Plan for emergent operative intervention."

Follow the hierarchy and ask for assistance. Always notify the upper level before making any critical interventions. Know your limit; if you are preparing to tackle a task for the first time, always call for backup to bring experience and safety to the scenario. The presence of senior/chief residents will also shield you from moments where others are critical of your decisions. Asking for help when tasks become overwhelming despite your best efforts at triaging and prioritizing is a sign of maturity and taking responsibility for patients.

You are never alone. Even if all other surgical residents appear to be occupied and unavailable, there are other healthcare providers in the hospital. Ask your ED colleague to help facilitate tasks such as line placements, start resuscitation, initiate antibiotic therapy, or call for critical consults such as cardiology for perioperative risk stratification. Be respectful and courteous to emergency department colleagues; they know how to reach just about every service in the hospital and will return the favor when you need their assistance.

Keep a sterile sharp instrument on hand. General surgery residents should be ready to wield a blade at a second's notice. Many reversible causes of acute life-threatening deterioration require invasive intervention, and no one should be more prepared to do so than you. Tension pneumothorax can be relieved merely by entering the thoracic cavity with a finger.

Finally, *remember to breathe* and always prepare for the worst-case scenario. If the surgeon in the room is panicking, so will everyone else. Take control of every battle and exude confidence through preparation and experience. The sun will always rise in the morning, and reinforcement will be here to relieve you of your duties.

Pearls
- Follow the chain of command and notify your upper level resident before making critical decisions or interventions. Senior residents bring experience and safety to foreign scenarios, which will protect you.
- Organize the chaos by maintaining a private electronic patient list in the EMR for call shifts. Include patients with pending tasks, new consults, and those with deteriorating clinical status.
- Actively think ahead to prepare for the worst-case scenario. In high-stress situations, others will naturally look to you for leadership and guidance. Remember to breathe and learn to keep a calm demeanor.
- Maintain a friendly relationship with your emergency room colleagues. They will appreciate your kind attitude and readily come to your aid when requested.
- Keep a sterile sharp instrument handy. Few things are more frustrating than opening up the sterile thoracotomy set and not having a blade for initial incision.
- Triage your patients and your tasks; always prioritize actions that advance patient care. Develop this skill to improve efficiency.
- Know your limit, and do not be afraid to ask for help when overwhelmed.

Chapter 13
Keeping Up with the Paperwork

Shelley Jain

Introduction

Paperwork is incredibly important in residency, and falling behind can create problems and hinder your progress or even graduation. Making a schedule and system to sit down to complete it all is very important. Whether it is a daily effort, weekly reminder, or monthly session, it is crucial that you find a paperwork system that works for you and stick to it for the next few years of residency.

Paperwork can be the bane of a surgical resident's existence. It seems never ending, but each one is incredibly important, from keeping yourself on track to correct documentation. At the end of residency, it is the paperwork that will document your progress and show your achievements. Residency success really is impossible without accurately logging your cases, getting the evaluations you need, and putting in the hours. Every resident forms their own system and rhythm to get it done, and it is up to you to find a consistent and successful one.

Duty Hours

Logging duty hours should be done weekly or monthly. Every residency has a system for logging duty hours, and it will usually be in the New Innovations application. Downloading the phone app and logging the hours daily when you enter and leave the hospital is one way. The alternative is to set aside time each week or month to log the hours on the online site. Setting a reminder to do this on a regular schedule is the best way to ensure that it is completed and accurate. You should log accurate

S. Jain (✉)
WellSpan Health, York, PA, USA
e-mail: sjain3@wellspan.org

hours and not be pressured to falsely report your hours. There will be certain hours to log for 24-h calls, clinic time, vacation time, etc., so it is important to be meticulous and report them truthfully.

Case Logs

The ACGME Case Log System is the only way to get credit for your cases in residency to count towards your minimum case logs required for graduation. This document is also one that should be completed regularly and carefully since you will be using this log as a reflection of your achievements and skills gained in your training. Using the mobile app to log cases as you complete them is a fast way to ensure that the logging is done accurately. Alternatively, you can use the online website to log cases for the week or the month. It is easy to fall behind on these logs, and going back to accurately represent which cases you have done can be time consuming and difficult. It is important to log the cases that you have participated in with the accurate designation as First Assist or Surgeon Junior or Chief. You will get credit to your minimum number of cases for only those cases that you are a surgeon junior or chief resident. It is frowned upon to have two residents log the same case, so if two residents did a significant portion of the same case, communicate before logging. If there are two separate portions of the case, they may be logged separately as two separate procedures. Logging these cases is essential to graduating surgical residency and proving that your experience was adequate in its breadth and depth.

Evaluations

Getting and giving evaluations each rotation you complete in residency are also time-sensitive paperwork that must be completed in residency. In person, mid-rotation, it is nice to get formative feedback from attendings, which can reflect in your written evaluations too. Make sure that your feedback is constructive and specific, and not too vague. Giving good timely feedback to peers and attendings on rotations is also important while you remember the experiences you have had in detail.

Personal Journaling

One great way to remember important case takeaways and interesting patients is to keep your own log (on an EMR) or a private notebook (in a HIPAA-safe manner) so that you can reference back to important teaching points. Our patients are our greatest teachers, and you will see hundreds in residency. To keep a log of ones that may be extra educational will be an asset as you become a chief and for oral boards.

Pearls
- Paperwork is incredibly important in residency; make sure that you have a schedule and system to complete it all.
- Log your duty hours regularly.
- Log your cases in the ACGME case log system after every case. You can use the mobile app to make it easy.
- Make sure that you regularly ask for and provide required evaluations that are constructive.

Chapter 14
Teaching Other Residents and Students

Benjamin A. Dixson and Emily O. Goddard

Every surgeon should strive to become an impactful teacher and to remain a lifelong learner. Teaching and passing on knowledge should be sprinkled throughout each and every day on the job. Even a small teaching moment, a short but rich educational pearl, may stick with a learner for a lifetime.

As a resident, teaching can be difficult due to the ever-increasing workload and narrowing time constraints. Each morning, the team must see all the patients, produce plans, put in orders, and then execute the plans, all before the operating room starts for the day. Sometimes, formal rounding is impossible. Sometimes, attendings round while residents are in the operating room with other attendings. How—and where—is there time for teaching? Well, unbelievably, there are plenty of opportunities. A surgery resident must be very aware and try not to rush through these opportunities for teaching when they present themselves throughout the stressful surgical day.

Teaching Other Residents and Students

There are many different scenarios during the average day in the life of a surgery resident where one can teach. Here are several settings where one can integrate teaching moments:

B. A. Dixson (✉)
ChristianaCare Health System, Newark, DE, USA
e-mail: benjamin.dixson@christianacare.org

E. O. Goddard
WellSpan Health, York, PA, USA

© The Author(s), under exclusive license to Springer Nature Switzerland AG 2023
A. Ratnasekera et al. (eds.), *General Surgery Residency Survival Guide*,
https://doi.org/10.1007/978-3-031-25617-2_14

- *Formal didactics*—Residents will often be invited to participate in formal clinical and/or didactic teaching sessions to students of all types and levels. These formal teaching roles can initially feel a bit daunting but try to put yourself in the learners' shoes. Try to recall what information you knew at their level, so that you may teach the appropriate level of information. Keep them engaged and ask questions; try to avoid strict lecturing.
- *Patient presentations*—Give feedback during and after oral patient presentations. Affirm things the medical student or resident did well (organization, pertinent information, etc.) and provide constructive direction on weaknesses.
- *Teach through imaging* —Take the time to review images (X-rays, CT scans, etc.) together. Try starting with what is normal in the image. Ask them what they see and then point out findings that you notice to be significant.
- *Operative case preparation*—Have an educational focus to review before a case. For example, read about the "critical view of safety" and anatomic variations for the laparoscopic cholecystectomy tomorrow. Setting targeted self-directed learning goals is key.
- *Surgical skills*—Be very mindful of your word choices and specific with direction. For example, while in the operating room performing laparoscopy, you may say "take your left hand and move it towards the patient's feet." When teaching a procedure or skill, demonstrate the technique while simultaneously describing it, and then have the student try themselves. "Show" and then have them "do."
- *Creating treatment plans* —Allow students and junior residents to create their own management plans for patients they see in the ED or in the clinic. It is especially important that these plans are always accompanied by discussion of a thorough differential diagnoses. Students and residents need to think through what the most likely diagnosis is and why, in order to fully understand the best treatment plan. Encouraging them to verbalize their diagnostic thought process and then treatment plan will allow them to grow both in their knowledge and confidence. This practice will lead to better clinical judgment later in residency.

It is important to keep in mind that each learner has his or her own unique learning style. To help each individual learner best, one should inquire and then tailor their teaching style to how the learner learns best. This ability to individually tailor one's teaching style can be immensely challenging but is the sign of a truly experienced educator. The more one can adapt their style of teaching, the more effective they will become.

Pearls
- Meet the learner where they are at. Engage them, inquire what they already know, understand about the topic at hand, and go from there. The Socratic method is not dead.
- Sharing even a small amount of knowledge or a simple concept or principle is often enough to demonstrate that you care about the education of those students/residents.
- Try to tailor the teaching style for each individual learner, and inquire what works best for them.

Chapter 15
Interactions with Nurses, OR, and Office Staff

James Juhng

Introduction

The hospital is a unique environment as a resident in comparison to a medical student. As a resident, you will be seen as an employee with responsibilities and provide guidance and information to help with the daily workflow. This includes the delicate work of hospital politics. The following members of the hospital are on your side to help care for patients before, during, and after surgery even if sometimes it does not feel like it. Assume that the staff has been working for more than 20 years and take their communication into consideration. Regardless of their behavior towards you, these are your teammates. If they are calling or paging, assume that they need your help!

Nurses

Nurses participate in all aspects of the hospital. They are linked to each other through you. In the emergency department (ED), new consults are first seen, and a plan is determined. The emergency department can become a very hectic environment, and closed-loop communication with the ED nurses establishes a few things. First, a disposition is established for the patient. Second, the patient's care is entrusted to you. Third, it helps build a reputation as a competent physician. If the patient needs admission, the next phase is the floor or intensive care unit (ICU). Floor nurses enjoy clarification. A page or a call is a request for help whether that is

J. Juhng (✉)
WellSpan Health, York, PA, USA
e-mail: jjuhng@wellspan.org

© The Author(s), under exclusive license to Springer Nature Switzerland AG 2023
A. Ratnasekera et al. (eds.), *General Surgery Residency Survival Guide*, https://doi.org/10.1007/978-3-031-25617-2_15

for clarification on an order, completing discharge paperwork, or bedside examination. ICU nurses enjoy intensity and puzzles. Their gut feeling is usually right. In the beginning, youwill be learning from them quite a bit. Their abilities to recognize morbid patterns are more right than wrong. But with some clinical experience mixed with basic science and critical thinking, you will be managing patient care in no time.

OR Staff

If the patient needs to go to the operating room (OR) from the ED or the floor, there are a number of characters you might encounter. The first is the circulating nurse and the scrub tech. These two individuals have met a lot of people and know when someone knows what they are doing. Be kind, be smart, and be well prepared. Good impressions with them usually help with subsequent cases. The next person is the charge nurse. They can help determine when the next case may go and provide an estimated time for upcoming surgeries. Anesthesia may be the anesthesiologist, the resident, or a certified registered nurse assistant. During the operation, please remember their name, as most have been labeled under the umbrella term "anesthesia."

Office Staff

Office staff often will have limited interaction with you. Depending on your institution, there may be a couple of diverse ways you will interact with office staff. The most common interaction is setting up outpatient follow-up. Usually, this is as simple as an email or a message through your home institution's electronic medical record. During clinic time, you will typically be with your attending. If you have a surgical resident run clinic, then your office staff will help schedule, call, and set up your patients.

Pearls
- Treat each nurse, surgical tech, and office staff member with respect for their experience and skills.
- Nurses are present at every aspect of a surgeon's life from the ED to the OR to the floor/ICU.

Chapter 16
Interactions with Residents and Attendings

James Juhng

Introduction

As a newly minted resident, there is an element of a corporate environment that is different than the years spent as a student. You will be dependent on your seniors to be leaders and guides when first starting. Your fellow juniors and interns will be colleagues who will help you make it through surgical residency.

Residents

Juniors The totem pole exists in medicine for a reason. Practicing medicine is difficult and takes years to build the experience and wisdom to make the right diagnosis and treatment plan. Instead of reinventing the wheel every year, textbooks, morbidity and mortality conferences, and the concept of graduated responsibility exist to transform a medical student into a surgeon. This will be the time to develop as a person capable of working on minimal sleep and maximal physical capacity, all while gaining as much knowledge and experience before all the responsibility lands on your shoulders. Be the dependable one. Learn from the mistakes of seniors and attendings and see how you can evolve through your interactions to become a future leader. Every surgeon is a leader, and it is only a matter of time until it is your turn to be one.

J. Juhng (✉)
WellSpan Health, York, PA, USA
e-mail: jjuhng@wellspan.org

63
A. Ratnasekera et al. (eds.), *General Surgery Residency Survival Guide*,
https://doi.org/10.1007/978-3-031-25617-2_16

Seniors Beginning residency may be difficult for several reasons. One of them is at the bottom of the totem pole every other resident outside intern year is your senior. There should always be respect when addressing seniors. They have already experienced an 80-h work-week intern year and are developing their clinical skills. With each year, there is a progressive adjustment in responsibility. A good, strong senior will do their best to make sure that attendings are happy while managing juniors and interns with tasks such as consults, consents, and progress notes. Sometimes, the managerial aspect is hard, but this will come with time and effort since leadership takes time and effort.

Attendings Interactions with attendings may initially be awkward given that their fund of knowledge far surpasses yours. However, within 3–4 years, working 80 hours a week while ideally studying 20 hours a week will build a foundation to have discussions about surgical pathology, procedures, and life. Throughout the years of working, presenting patients will become easier, having a thought-out differential and diagnosis, and the surgical skills to back it up. Attendings in turn will see you either as a dependable individual or as someone they must deal with until you graduate. Be knowledgeable and dependable in order to reach the goal of junior attending by PGY-5 year, and eventually you will be speaking as peers.

Pearls
- Respect the totem pole between juniors and seniors. Juniors should expect to learn from the experience and wisdom of seniors when it comes to knowledge and workload. Seniors should expect to learn how to manage people and events to become a leader.
- Attendings are future peers, and it is only a matter of time until you get there. The goal is to learn enough surgery to be seen as an acting junior attending PGY-5 and as a fellow.

Chapter 17
Curbside Consultation

Ellen Pekar

The curbside consult is a prevalent situation in the collegial world of medicine. It holds a unique medicolegal role and has become widespread in medicine.

"Hey! Can I ask you a question about this patient we have down in the ED?" or "Hello I have some imaging I wanted to run by you" are some of the calls you will inevitably receive as a physician.

The curbside consult is an informal consult from one clinician to another clinician currently uninvolved with the care of the patient in question. A curbside consult is more limited in scope and depth than a formal consultation. Legally, there is no medical liability for a curbside consult as the liability for medical malpractice is based on an existing doctor-patient relationship [1]. There are however some exceptions to the above rule: (1). Per the Emergency Medical Treatment and Active Labor Act, any interaction between an emergency department physician and an on-call physician regarding an ED patient is legally not a curbside consult. (2). A physician who covers for a colleague assumes full medical and legal responsibility for their colleagues' patients. (3). An interaction between a resident and an attending physician cannot constitute a curbside consult as the attending physician is responsible for the staff they supervise [1].

The question becomes: why one should participate in a curbside consult? Medicine historically has bred a collaborative and collegial environment. The act of seeking a second opinion via curbside consult can expedite patient care, provide different viewpoints on patient's care, and strengthen relationships with other physicians.

When receiving a curbside consult, one must first determine whether the consult would be better served as a formal consultation [2]. A formal consultation may be more appropriate on a more complex patient who would require examination and

E. Pekar (✉)
WellSpan Health, York, PA, USA
e-mail: epekar@wellspan.org

A. Ratnasekera et al. (eds.), *General Surgery Residency Survival Guide*, https://doi.org/10.1007/978-3-031-25617-2_17

thorough review before rendering an opinion. A formal consultation may also be more appropriate than a curbside consult if you are being consulted for your specialization or expertise in an area [3]. If the decision is made to perform a curbside consult, the consulting physician may provide their opinion but should not place orders or change existing orders. Documentation is a tricky issue. If one is seeking a curbside consultation, they should try to avoid documenting the consulting physician's name unless permitted so by the consulting physician. If one is performing the consultation, it is up to their discretion to document their consultation.

Pearls
- A curbside consult is an informal consult from one clinician to another uninvolved with the care of the patient in question.
- A curbside consultation between the emergency department and the on-call physician is legally not possible under EMTALA.
- Curbside consults can expedite patient care, provide different viewpoints in patient care, and enhance professional relationships.
- When receiving an informal consultation, the first decision to make is whether the consult would be better served as a formal consultation. Then carry out the consultation and make the decision of whether documentation is necessary.
- Documentation of the curbside consult is up to the discretion of the consulting physician.

References

1. Cotton V. Legal risks of "Curbside" consults. Am J Cardiol. 2010;106(1):135–8.
2. Kuo D. Curbside consultation practices and attitudes among primary care physicians and medical subspecialists. JAMA. 1998;280(10):905.
3. Psychiatry (Edgemont). Curbside Consultations. 2010;7(5):51–3.

Part III
Life Outside of Work/Finances

Chapter 18
Finding Love in Residency

India Jones

There is no mistaking that surgical residency can be grueling. I find it redundant to belabor such a well-known point. But what is consistently understated is what it is exactly that makes it so grueling. It is everything outside of the hospital walls—finding and maintaining things that are important to you.

The summer after my intern year, we got engaged. There was this kind, intelligent, and caring man that had the audacity to ask us (me and my career) to build a life with him. He went through bounds secretly searching through my call schedule to figure out a weekend that I was off, and finally found a weekend that worked for our family and friends to ask me to marry him.

During my intern year of residency, I was certain that our relationship would suffer some setbacks. We were in two separate cities; I was a resident, and he was a medical student applying for residency. Every weekend that I had off, he would drive hours for us to spend 1 day together. (I'm not sure how much of the time we spent together counts for anything valuable, given I was always falling asleep since I was so exhausted from work.) But he was patient. And he was understanding.

He and I first became friends in medical school. Although we went to the same school, we first met at a "med student mixer" that included all the schools in the area—it was a busy event. When he asked to buy me a drink, we were surprised to realize we went to the same med school and soon after began to grow an honest and intimate friendship.

Towards the end of the medical school, we started to transition our friendship into something more serious, and the strife of surgical residency truly put our intentions with each other to the test. When you are working close to 80 h/week, it is very difficult to have energy for anything other than your basic needs. That is why it is

I. Jones (✉)
Cooper University Hospital, Camden, NJ, USA
e-mail: Jones-india@cooperhealth.edu

© The Author(s), under exclusive license to Springer Nature
Switzerland AG 2023
A. Ratnasekera et al. (eds.), *General Surgery Residency Survival Guide*,
https://doi.org/10.1007/978-3-031-25617-2_18

absolutely vital to have a flexible partner that is able to find a place in your busy life without it becoming extensively laborious for you.

I think the key in finding the type of love worth having as a surgical resident is being completely authentic and honest in your dating endeavors. First, you need to be honest with yourself, about your desires, needs, and expectations, and secondly, you need to be honest with whoever you share your time with. Sure, my fiancé and I met in medical school, but I was able to date in both medical school and early in my residency. I was always open and transparent about what my life and free time looked like, regardless of the seriousness of the romantic endeavor at the time. People have a right to know what they are signing up for, and I was serious about my right to be picky about who I allowed in my life. Your free time becomes so much more valuable when you do not have a lot of it. Whether you are dating for friendship, for a serious relationship, or for fun, less time is wasted, and more parties are fulfilled when honesty and transparency are utilized.

I was fortunate to have done my medical school and residency training in major metropolitan areas. There was never a shortage of diverse professionals, and especially medical professionals. I find this to be a positive thing, although some of my other friends absolutely abhor the thought of dating another medical professional. I find solace in "talking shop" with my partner after a long day, and his understanding and relating to my ranting. Others would find this to be redundant and excessive. This debate is not a matter of right or wrong, but a matter of truthful examination of your own desires and values.

My partner has since matriculated into anesthesiology residency in the same city as me, and we were able to move in together as we began our union. We found that both of us being in medicine made it much easier to gain a shared sense of understanding as a couple. He knew first-hand what it was like for me. But that did not mean we did not have challenges.

How do you manage when two people in a relationship are exhausted, burnt out, crabby, and irritable when they get home? How do you interact with each other? How do you determine who supports who, and who gets prioritized when you are both equally spent? It becomes a lot.

We owe a huge amount of our success as a couple to outsourcing, planning, and flexibility. Instead of arguing about whose turn it is to do laundry, we learned to hire a housekeeper every month who deep cleans and does all our house tasks. Each week we take turns meal-prepping, so we are not burdened with figuring out what is for dinner every night. And sometimes, even with all the planning in the world, flexibility and sacrifice are required. If one person is obviously more stressed than the other, whether it be for an exam, deadline, or life event, the other person steps in and carries the burden of the household tasks in support of the other. Shared responsibility for each other's wellness is invaluable.

Another key in both finding and maintaining love in residency is intention! Making time for love is so important. I think it should be emphasized how vast "love" is, and how it encompasses not only romantic love, but also love in friendship, family, other relationships, and love with yourself. Love is something that must be cultivated and actively worked on. Make time to call your parents every week. Invite your friends to visit you on a weekend off. If you are looking for romantic interests, go out on a date once a month. Speak to interesting people you meet at the grocery store, gym, or kickball club. Get a massage once a month or treat yourself to your favorite restaurant. Love requires intention and commitment; an intentional space must be created for it because residency will not do it for you.

There is no manual or blueprint for finding love in residency, but there is one overarching fact—we must be as serious and as zealous with cultivating the various embodiments of love in our lives as we are about becoming exceptional surgeons. When we do this, we become more fulfilled, empathetic, and emotionally intelligent human beings and thus even better surgeons for our patients.

Pearls
- Determine whether you are interested in a partner who is in healthcare; we spend a majority of our time here, and a lot of people first meet their partners in a work setting.
- Honesty and transparency are pivotal, both with yourself and with your loved ones; it will help you set realistic expectations about what you can contribute to a relationship as a resident and what you expect in a relationship.
- Pairing is your friend: call your loved ones while driving, cooking, or walking on the treadmill; there are small pockets of time throughout the day that can be harvested.
- There will be periods of time where you have nothing to contribute to a relationship and that is totally okay; it is important that your loved ones understand this.
- Be clear with your loved ones about how they can support you through this journey.

Chapter 19
Relationships: How to Keep Your Significant Other Happy

Heather Geist and Puja D. Patel

What makes a successful relationship in residency? One of the million-dollar residency questions. Depending on when you met your significant other, they could be following you from medical school to residency to fellowship or meeting you somewhere in between. It is impossible to accurately predict our next move, and we sit in hopes that our loved one will follow us as we follow our dreams. Some of us are committed to other physicians and others, to people who could never fully understand the stress we endure on a daily basis. Why a "golden weekend" is really just a normal weekend and why we have to schedule vacations one year in advance. We are not able to commit to last-minute plans or sometimes (many times) even be home for dinner. We hope that they will be willing to understand our schedules, our stress, and our absence.

So, you are with another physician? That is great! The only problem is, they are not in surgery and still do not understand why we work the amount we do. They ask, "wow, what specialty was so terrible they actually had to cap the work week to 80 hours?!" We meekly raise our hands, "Um. Well, it was probably because of surgery."

Okay, so none of this applies to you because you are with another surgeon? Now you are struggling with aligning the "golden weekends" which are few and far between. Who is on a 24 hour shift this time? When will we see our spouse next? It will be worth it, right?

The answer is; yes. You see, many of us cannot imagine doing anything else. All you can hope is that you find someone who can appreciate this fact and support your dreams. We do have to give a little though. Do I dare say it? It is not all about us after all! If they can support us, we must support them. We must remember the obstacles

H. Geist (✉) · P. D. Patel
Lehigh Valley Health Network, Allentown, PA, USA
e-mail: Heather.Geist@lvhn.org; Puja.Patel@lvhn.org

© The Author(s), under exclusive license to Springer Nature
Switzerland AG 2023
A. Ratnasekera et al. (eds.), *General Surgery Residency Survival Guide*,
https://doi.org/10.1007/978-3-031-25617-2_19

they face by being our partner, and let us be honest, there are many. From something as big as uprooting their whole life to as simple as not being able to go to dinner with their spouse on a whim. They scroll through social media, seeing their friends traveling with their significant other and are probably thinking, "I wish we could do that." Residency is a bigger commitment than we could have imagined, but we are here to tell you, it is possible to be in a happy and healthy relationship during surgical residency. It just takes effort and the right person.

Puja's Story

My life was going as planned. I had a boyfriend with whom an engagement ring was purchased and ready for my finger. He was finishing up his MBA, and I was finishing up my second year of medical school, ready to take USMLE Step 1 and move onto a lighter schedule with clinical rotations. We were long distance, and I was so caught up in my education that I did not see the red flags. When he asked me, "Are you sure you don't want to do family medicine instead? It's much shorter and the hours are better," I laughed it off. Most weekends together were spent studying, and I refused to make time for any plans that would interfere with my tight study schedule. My dreams were set in stone. I was going to be a surgeon, no matter what it takes! At the time, I did not realize the damage that commitment was causing to my personal life. One week before my USMLE Step 1, I Facetimed him as I did every night. He said the famous last words, "I can't do this anymore." Just like that, my perfectly planned life was no more. The timing could not have been worse, but I decided to mentally block out the conversation and continue to study for next week. After my test, I concluded two important things. First, I would no longer waste tears or time on people who did not support my lifelong dreams. Second, I was partially if not mostly to blame for the failure of our relationship. Though I know he was not right for me and would never have accepted my career as a surgeon, the latter was still hard to swallow.

I met my husband in my third year of medical school. He is not in medicine, but I made sure early on that he knew what he was getting into. I love my husband, and he is perfect in every way. He supports my dreams, no matter how big. If I say, "I'm thinking of doing 5-year fellowship 1000 miles away," he is my biggest cheerleader. You may say, "Why are you even answering this question? Why are you writing this chapter? You don't even know the struggle!" Sorry, one detail I left out. I forgot to mention that my husband did not move to residency with me. Instead, he stayed at his job and has been visiting any weekend I am not on call. When I opened my envelope on match day, my overwhelming excitement was quickly coated with dread. I knew the reality. I wanted to follow my dreams but not at the expense of his own, so I happily compromised with my husband. I miss him every day he is not here, but I know this is what works for us. If he had left his job to move with me, he would be unhappy and that was not acceptable to me. Even though he says that he would have moved, I know that he would have resented me and the failure of our relationship would have been inevitable. I was never one to compromise in the past. It was all about my goals, but with him, that change felt effortless. We support each other every day, and there is no one else I would rather experience this journey with.

So, my advice? Try not to compare yourself to others and do not let anyone tell you that you are not doing right by your significant other, especially if you both are happy. What works for us may not work for someone else and that is okay. There will be compromises; it is inevitable, but the key is to find someone with whom you are willing to make those compromises with. Make decisions together, show them they are appreciated, and always make time for them. The right person will support you just as you support them, and it should not feel like a sacrifice. Communication is everything, and it is vital that they know you hear them. My husband and I do not see each other every day, but whether it is on our drive home from work or right before bed, we always make time for each other to talk. Listen to their hardships from the day. Though they may pale in comparison to ours which may have consisted of the death of a patient, we should not imply that their day was not as bad as ours. Give them your time. It is the least we can do.

Heather's Story

Life is messy and sometimes so are relationships. Residency puts the ultimate stress test on relationships—with significant others, family, and friends. And it is not just surgical residency that pushes people to their limits. My previous fiancé was also in medicine, an internal medicine resident that was experiencing 24–28 hour calls for the first time, the death and illness of patients, and the struggle of continuing to learn the wealth of information before him. I was finishing up my fourth year of medical school, bright eyed at the next chapter of my professional career and being able to start our life together, with medicine being one of our many common threads. We kept a very open communication channel, often discussing each other's medical stories, experiences, and hardships. I felt that our relationship was strong and he often agreed. We made time for fun away from the books and study materials. What I did not realize is how much my fiancé's work was weighing on him. In a matter of a week, our lives changed (two weeks before my match day). The stress of work became too much that he was exhausted and withdrawn, doing what he could to make it through his days feeling riddled with anxiety. We were not living together and were two hours apart, which felt like 1000 miles with how busy our work schedules were. And then it happened. On a cold winter day, he did not show up to work and was not answering phone calls. I had just talked to him the night before. As I drove to his apartment, I had one of those gut feelings you just know; before I even got into my car, I felt like I knew. I arrived to the police, an ambulance, and one of his work colleagues. He was dead.

Just like that, my life deflated around me. I was about to start the hardest stretch of my professional career and life without my greatest support, my fellow doctor with whom I shared an understanding of the hardships surrounding us both. There are so many details of these moments that could fill a book alone. Each day was a chance to move forward, and slowly I did. Looking back at this transition, my greatest takeaway is that if life throws you a curveball, be honest with yourself about the time and space you need. When you are ready, you will know. No one writes the rule book on life.

After I took the time I needed for me, I found myself open and ready to see if there was another someone out there for me. Here enters the horrible world of dating in residency. When you spend about 80 hours a week within the hospital walls, it leaves very little time for finding a human outside of medicine. I always swore I would never use dating apps. I was skeptical. It seemed time consuming and superficial, and I had no idea when I would have time to go on dates. But thanks to the encouragement of some of my friends, I finally joined a couple dating site when I resolved to the fact I was not going to meet anybody if I did not embrace it. I went on a few dates, but nothing worth spending a second date on. We all know our time is precious, and I was not about to sacrifice my hours outside of the hospital on someone who was intimidated by the idea of a female surgeon, could not keep up with an intellectual conversation, or was not willing to learn about what dating life with a surgical resident would look like. I knew what I would need and decided I was not willing to sacrifice in certain areas of my relationship and life. The requirements were plenty, and the standards were high. I felt like I would never find someone who could understand my work-life, let alone what had happened in my previous relationship.

I proved myself wrong and one evening after a very long day at work hopped on a video chat date (you know, the whole Covid pandemic thing …). And from that day on, my (new) fiancé and I have worked to foster a relationship in the wild world of surgical residency. I found it very important to let him know what surgical residency truly was—no sugarcoating. Expectations had to be clear of my schedule and commitment. One of the things I admire about my fiancé is that he did everything he could to try to understand my world, and while he knows he never fully can, he is an incredibly good listener. It is a daily two-way street—making little sacrifices for each other. We each make a point to notice the little things we do for each other, because we know it is not always easy for the other person. The bottom line is dating in residency is hard—it takes time and commitment and most importantly communication. Do not sacrifice yourself for your relationship. And when you know what you want, stay true to that because it makes the someone you find that much more meaningful.

Pearls
- Ensure that your partner recognizes the difficulty of surgical residency: the long hours, the 24 hour shifts, and the endless studying. It is our life's work and we are proud of our accomplishment, so it is important that your partner understands this.

- Support is a two-way street. They support you and in turn we should support them.
- Make time for your partners. It is the least we can do for everything they do for us.
- Everyone's experience is different and do not compare yourself to another couple. What works for you may not work for others and that is fine, as long as you and your partner are happy.

Chapter 20
How to Maintain Personal Relationships

Nadj L. Pierre

Finding and keeping love while training as a general surgery resident is a balancing act. Thankfully, the field has evolved and made it possible for residents to strive for work-life balance. With the push towards specialization and the higher attrition rates, programs have started listening to residents in order to maintain recruitment but also retention [1]. Home life is undeniably linked to job satisfaction, so how we choose to spend our time outside the hospital ultimately affects how we perform in the operating room [2]. I have found that there are five cardinal rules when entertaining the idea of a love life while being a resident.

Plan

When dating, planning is useful. Figure out what you are looking for, hedonia or eudaimonia. That is, pleasure or fulfillment … or both? There is no wrong answer, assuming that you know which one you are pursuing. If you are like Aristotle, you might believe that because humans can reason, pleasure alone cannot be the answer. If you are like Oscar Wilde, you may align more with getting rid of temptation by yielding to it. When you know why you have decided to be with someone in residency, it makes planning more purposeful. What you do with the golden weekends and the post-call days is paramount. This also reveals who you want to be in your life. Your free time is precious. Spend it wisely.

N. L. Pierre (✉)
WellSpan Health, York, PA, USA
e-mail: npierre2@wellspan.org

Be Open-Minded

Accept that no one will understand completely what you are going through, except maybe another surgical resident. Stop thinking that people are crazy, stupid, or evil when you disagree with them. Exercise thoughtful disagreement: do not try to convince the other party that you are right; instead, find out why they think their view is true and decide what to do about it. Understand that you might never understand and come to terms with that.

Forgive People

This is about accepting the things you cannot change because relinquishing control is where true freedom lies. The therapeutic model breaks it down in four Rs: Responsibility, Remorse, Restoration, and Renewal. Lastly, it is about accepting yourself and all your shortcomings. Because even general surgery residents fall short sometimes.

Say Thank You

Residency is taxing, both physically and psychologically. Remember to thank your partner because, although they might not be a surgical resident pulling 80-h weeks, they still chose to be in this with you. Saying "thank you" gives you more energy and vitality. You fall asleep quicker and stay asleep longer. Systolic blood pressure decreases, and you are overall more relaxed and less depressed. That sets you up for being a better person and partner.

Do Good

Do not confuse doing good with doing no harm. Do no harm is the bare minimum. It is the oath you take in medical school to practice non-maleficence. You must seek out good. Little acts of kindness go a long way. Saying thank you is well paired with acts of service. Take out the trash even if you are tired. Pick up the mail on your way in from night shift. Exhausted, but pursuing.

Remember that good relationships make for a good life. The people you allow in your life during these trying five plus years matter. Figure out who you want that to be and take good care of them because they are also making a sacrifice.

Pearls
- Maintaining relationships requires you to put in some work through acts of kindness, planning, forgiveness, and showing appreciation.
- Relationships during residency are hard, but not impossible.
- Understanding the needs of other people in your life and balancing how to meet those needs are important.

References

1. Sullivan MC, Yeo H, Roman SA, Bell RH Jr, Sosa JA. Striving for work-life balance: effect of marriage and children on the experience of 4402 US general surgery residents. Ann Surg. 2013;257(3):571–6.
2. Carter JV, Polk HC Jr, Galbraith NJ, McMasters KM, Cheadle WG, Poole M, Galandiuk S. Women in surgery: a longer term follow-up. Am J Surg. 2018;216(2):189–93.

Chapter 21
Motherhood and Residency

Jane Stevens

Atul Gawande has 5 rules for surgeons. Make a connection with your patients, do not complain, count something (do some sort of research even if it is just your own patients), remember to change (do not get stuck in the way you have always done it), and finally, most importantly, remember to write something.

Here, I am going to start with Rule #5. I am going to write something. They say to start with what you know. What do I know? I know surgical residency. I know what it is like to be a woman in surgery, and more than that, I know what it is like to be a mom in residency.

Dr. Gawande's five rules are meant to be some advice given from an experienced surgeon to a novice surgeon. Especially with Rule #5, he means that there is fulfillment and enlightenment to be gained within the difficult world of medicine by simply writing things down. The sharing of experiences and struggles of being a resident I think can be helpful and useful for other residents to read about. The act of sharing and of receiving experiences is beneficial on both ends. The sharing of it into a community of other residents and physicians helps us not to feel so alone and isolated. The act of opening up our lived experiences can be therapeutic, as well as reading about someone else's experience especially in parallel to our own can be bolstering and strengthening.

Full disclosure: I am a surgical resident. I would say, is one of the most rigorous and longer residencies. We have very long hours and high expectations. Most surgical residents spend 5–8 years in residency. Compared to our colleagues in some other specialties, that is a very long time. Residency is hard. The stamina it takes to work hour after hour to be, oftentimes, "low man" and never to be the master of a job can be wearing and frustrating. The 80 hour workweeks, fatigue, and lack of

J. Stevens (✉)
Oregon Health and Science University, Portland, OR, USA
e-mail: stevjane@ohsu.edu

© The Author(s), under exclusive license to Springer Nature
Switzerland AG 2023
A. Ratnasekera et al. (eds.), *General Surgery Residency Survival Guide*,
https://doi.org/10.1007/978-3-031-25617-2_21

personal time can be alternatively soul crushing and unsatisfying. Our lives become those of our patients and their families, often without thoughts of our own. There is a lot of giving and not a lot of getting.

Additionally, I am a parent. My kids were in elementary school when I started this process with medical school, and now as I am in my fourth year of residency, they are 18 and 20 years old.

Parenting is hard, especially after a long day in the hospital. It is very much like having two jobs, and your second job starts when you walk in the house at the end of a long day (or in the morning after working all night): never-ending laundry, meals to prepare, and kids to catch up with. For me, the 'catching up with' part happens continuously. I have checked grades at work, given pep talks at work, and scolded at work. I am available by phone most of the time. I am always the mom. I am always on the job, no matter where I am, worrying about them and carrying the mental load (the ongoing mental planning/involvement/attention to detail that most mothers do) of being their mother—all the time.

Many of us do have children, and if not yet, then another difficult decision looms, the 'when' of it. When is the right time? Especially for women, this becomes a decision fraught with interpersonal conflict. Job or family? And how do I have both while continuing to dedicate myself to the field I have spent my whole adult life working towards?

A fellow recently told a group of residents I was with that we would 'be either good parents or good residents, but not both.' My initial reaction was how can that be true? He felt like he was a neglectful father because he was a good resident, and my first thought was 'well you're a man so of course you have a choice.' I am sure that is sexist of me. But I do feel that for most families, there are differences in the roles for mom vs. dad. I don't feel like I have a choice to be an absentee mom. At the end of the day I need to be present and available for my kids, even if I am not available in person. As a mom and a resident, I do not feel I can sacrifice either role. I think part of what makes me a good resident is the fact that I am a good parent as well. So many skills in medicine are honed with parenting: for example, patience, perseverance, authority, strength, and understanding—all developed in the raising of children and applied to the caring of patients.

So, what do I do to survive being a parent as well as a resident? OK, let us get to the secret. Well, there is no secret. Only life before and life after having kids. Except that life after looks a lot different as a resident. As best you can, you merge worlds that seem incompatible. Most of us do it quietly with little complaint. The fact that we do it while being parents is for the most part underappreciated and under-recognized. I think this dual role should be celebrated. It is a challenge to deal with sick patients, emergent patients while also coping with whatever is going on at home, a sick child, an issue at school, perhaps behavioral issues. Multi-tasking is essential.

I heard a female surgeon speak about learning to be a surgeon and managing household duties. She said that anyone who is training to be a surgeon or practicing surgery should not also be cleaning the bathtub. That spoke to me at the time. I was struggling to complete my first years in residency while spending a lot of my mental load on whether the toilets had been cleaned that week. I felt like I was failing in every way if my house was a mess even if I was managing at work. After a few tear-filled discussions with my husband… who I must say would totally jump up and clean the toilet if I asked him to … what came out is that we just are not wired the same way. He does not carry around in his head all the things I am thinking/worrying about daily. Like all my mental tabs are open, all the time. So back to the breakdown—after confessing this added mental burden of feeling like I was failing at home as a housekeeper (not to mention as a mother and wife), we decided that the best plan for us as a family would be to hire house cleaners. I would not say that is the answer for everyone, and I am conscious of the financial cost, but honestly it helped a tremendous amount with the mental load I was carrying. I know without a doubt that once a week, no matter what else is happening, the toilets are clean! For you, maybe it's not the toilet, maybe it's a bedtime story, or making sure they have healthy snacks at school. Will some planning and support, surgical moms can find solutions to problems that seem incompatible with residency. Maybe read the bedtime story over facetime at a set time. Maybe plan out the weeks' healthy snacks on your day off. Or recruit a trusted family or friend to step into your role when needed, whether at a parent-teacher conference or soccer practice. Sometimes it really does take a village.

I do not know many that are as lucky as I am when it comes to partners, but my husband is one of the most patient and understanding. It is obvious that I would have struggled a lot more in residency had it not been for his solid and unwavering support and understanding. We have had to negotiate "money talk" and have made an effort not to describe our money as his or mine (my sad, low low income). We come at it as a team with the common goal of getting through residency successfully. Ultimately, it is a tough road. It takes stamina, grit, and resilience. I look forward to vacations a great deal, mostly so I can sleep. My kids are OK. Above all, I know that they are proud of me. They have seen their mom do a really hard thing and survive. They have seen that there is no 'I can't' or 'I'm not smart enough.' That it is about hard work all the way. Sometimes, I have thought about 'what is wrong with me that I went down this road.' Mostly, I want to be really good at something. I want my life to have as much meaning as possible. Like when I applied to nursing school all those years ago, "I just want to help people."

Indeed, it must be mentioned that I would not be able to do this if I was not partnered with a man who has supported us in every way the whole way through. That would be the secret I think, choosing to be with someone who can be selfless and forgiving, and willing to undergo a 'residency' of their own, in the role of chief supporter and cheerleader. Our relationship has grown and evolved as I have been a resident. He is willing to suffer the long absences, stress, and work hours, with our eye on the final destination and what our lives will be like at the end of this journey. Our kids are OK, I bond with them, and I make sure that I am still mostly available when they need me, even if only by phone. Right now, it is quality time over quantity of time that remains important. We are all trying to get through and survive the experience of residency. It's a long road and I am no expert for sure. But how lucky am I to have kids like mine? Successful and loving, they are people enjoy hanging out with, surely that is every mother's goal.

Pearls
- Make quality time over quantity of time with your children.
- Remain available for them emotionally if only by phone.
- Stay engaged and involved in any way you can, and keep track of what is happening.
- Save your off time for meaningful interactions with them, not housework!
- Lean on your spouse and others and make residency a family goal.

Chapter 22
Parenthood in Residency

Babak S. Sadri and Steven J. Capece

Introduction

Two fathers, one stay-at-home mother and one who works outside of the home, all with unique challenges. All who attempt to find balance and navigate the trials of residency and parenthood. None who would trade in their positions for anything in the world. This brief chapter, split into two parts, attempts to describe the experiences of both.

Parenthood in Residency: Part 1

Babak S. Sadri

Residency training is a taxing time period, not only for the resident, but also for their families. Having children can only add to the ever-growing responsibilities of the resident. However, many residents enter residency already having had children, or decide to have children during residency. There are several tools that can help residents manage responsibilities of being a parent and a resident while being mindful of their own well-being, as well as the well-being of those around them:

1. Have an open discussion with your partner about your mutual goals. Your partner's support throughout your journey is key.
2. Ask for help from family/friends.
3. Communicate with your colleagues/residency program and plan ahead of time.

B. S. Sadri (✉) · S. J. Capece
Lehigh Valley Health Network, Allentown, PA, USA
e-mail: Babak.Sadri@lvhn.org; Steven.Capece@lvhn.org

© The Author(s), under exclusive license to Springer Nature
Switzerland AG 2023
A. Ratnasekera et al. (eds.), *General Surgery Residency Survival Guide*,
https://doi.org/10.1007/978-3-031-25617-2_22

4. Carry your share of duties in residency. Others should not pay the price for your life choices.
5. Time management is key. You will be sleeping less … much less than an average resident.
6. Involve your kids in your errands (picking up mail, grocery).
7. Do not try to be a perfectionist parent. Understand and accept that there will be sacrifices.

The decision to have kids was mutual and well thought out by both my wife and I who had already been married for several years and did not want to wait any longer until the "right time." We were both wedding photographers before my journey in medicine began. Once I started medical school, she continued to shoot and help manage our photography business as I had less and less time. I knew I wanted to become a surgeon and had an open discussion with her, who as usual was supportive of me regardless of the tough road ahead. But now we both wanted kids and felt that there would never be a perfect time to do this with all of our responsibilities. Waiting for the "right time" in our case would not just be for a year or two as my surgical training and fellowship could take up to 8 or more years, and we decided we would be too old by then.

We had our first daughter in my third year of medical school. After she was born, my wife took a break from working in order to care for her. We realized we had to make sacrifices from the beginning. We downscaled our business, and I took out more student loans to cover the living expenses. Fortunately, during medical school, I had enough time to spend with my daughter and help out my wife since we had no family around to help.

However, things changed significantly during residency. I was working for long hours and not always around to help. We did however want our daughter to have a sibling, and we did not want a large age gap between the two. So, we planned our second daughter towards the end of my intern year in surgery. This was also a mutual decision and with the understanding that there would need to be even more sacrifices than our first experience. Financial issues, although still present, were not as significant now that I had an income from residency, so we could allocate less and less time to our photography business. Once we found out about pregnancy, I had an open discussion with my residency program leaders and co-residents and planned appropriately. I remember I was on call when my wife went into labor. She drove herself to the hospital. I am ashamed to admit but I recall being forced by my co-residents and attendings to leave my shift and spend time with her. I am glad I took their advice because she gave birth 3 h later. She has been gracious enough to never hold that against me to this date. I took 5 days of leave to help her and returned back to work once my father arrived in town to help. Both my wife and I understood that having kids in residency is a personal choice, and we did not wish for my colleagues to be burdened by our decision more than they already were.

Fast-forward a few years, and I am now proud of what my wife and I have been through and accomplished together. I have learned many things about myself as a parent and a physician in training. As cliché as it sounds, during residency, time management is key. Although not always possible, especially in a surgical residency, I try to set aside an hour each night to play with my kids. I include them in activities or errands that I already have to do: I take them for a walk to check the mail or to buy groceries. We may even stop by for an ice cream on the way. Sometimes, they may already be asleep, but I find that they are usually more than happy to wake up and step outside for a little while to stargaze with me, especially if I have not seen them for a few days.

In retrospect, the past few years have been some of the most challenging of our married life. Nonetheless, those challenges have not been impossible to overcome with the right mindset. It is important to avoid being a perfectionist. We made our decision to have kids knowing that there would be challenges and frustrations along the way. We realized that we would be imperfect parents, and we were perfectly fine with that. I have occasionally made the mistake of comparing myself to other parents who have the luxury of more time and energy for their kids; however, I quickly reason my way out of this pitfall. I may not have been as present in the lives of my children as much as I had hoped for, but I keep reminding myself that this is only temporary, and I am striving to make a better future for them. I recall all the instances that I have been there for them despite being exhausted. I may not have been a perfect parent, but I have been good enough, and that thought is enough to keep me on track.

Although having kids in residency has been very challenging—and I wholeheartedly blame my children for my receding hairline rather than the stresses of a surgical training—for me the bittersweet realization is that they bring me more joy and purpose in life than ever before, despite all of their challenges.

Parenthood in Residency: Part 2

Steven J. Capece

Intern year is a time filled with uncertainty and second guessing. As I transitioned into being a "real" doctor, I felt as if things could not become more challenging, but life has a way of throwing curveballs at you. My wife and I had been together since we were teenagers and were heading into our second year of marriage. We were eager to have a baby, but apprehensive. When would the right time present itself? Knee deep into intern year, the right time seemed more like a fallacy than a reality.

Amid night shifts and seemingly never-ending calls, we found out that my wife was pregnant in the second half of my first year—just as I was really mastering my role as intern. An excited shriek beaconed me into the next room as my wife revealed a pregnancy test with two prominent lines. Positive? Could it be? Amazing, how drastically life changes from one second to another. That night, my wife and I could barely sleep, trying to wrap our heads around how we would manage. Unbelievable joy mixed with utter terror.

It took a week, but we started piecing together how we would tackle parenthood in this stage of our lives. She was a newly licensed attorney; we were both treading water and figuring out our new roles professionally. The idea of raising a baby while our family, and only support system, was over 1500 miles away provided an extra stress. Could anyone fly up for the birth? How much time would I be able to take off for my child's birth? Would my wife have to face this alone? If I felt guilt for being away so much before, it instantaneously doubled.

I was candid with program leadership and my fellow residents about our growing family. Although it felt uncomfortable to voice my desire to take time off after my child's birth, I was able to piece together 2 weeks' off around the time my wife was to deliver. My program leadership and fellow residents were understanding about allowing me to be there for milestone appointments.

The next few months, my limited free time was dedicated to slowly piecing together a nursery, researching the best baby products, and taking some first-time parenting classes. How was there so much that I did not know? We did our Covid-friendly virtual gender reveal with all of our friends and family over Zoom. Pink confetti filled our living room while a combination of shocked and excited faces screamed out through our laptop, "It's a girl!" As if overnight, the nursery became much pinker and flower filled.

Nine months flew by as it tends to when working as a surgery resident. The saying "the days are long but the years are short" comes to mind. Before I knew it, I was leaving the hospital on Friday evening and starting my 2 weeks' off for paternity leave. My wife and I had one last final weekend to get the final few things in order before her induction on Friday. After a hard rotation with limited free time, I was looking forward to one last weekend just me and my wife when … Crash. One totaled car and a very pregnant wife picking her husband up from the side of the road was more labor inducing than any amount of Pitocin. After about a 24-h labor ending in C-section and a 6-h NICU stay in a hospital I was far too familiar with, our baby was here.

The remainder of my paternity leave was filled with doing everything I could to support my trooper of a wife, knowing that soon I would be back to my resident schedule. It went quick, and soon I started the process of trying to manage residency and fatherhood. Most days were filled with working all day to coming home and changing diapers, cleaning bottles/pump supplies, bath time, etc. I don't think I have ever been so physically exhausted trying to manage both of my positions.

A new curveball came when my wife had to return to her job as a criminal defense attorney with a close to an hour commute. The transition to daycare was hard, knowing that no one will care for your baby like you will. The first few weeks of daycare were tough. My wife would cry, and I felt helpless. What could I say or do to make it better? My only advice for those in a similar position is to give you and your partner a lot of grace during the transition. It is hard to give your baby up for someone else to care for, but it gets better over time and soon everyone will adjust to the change. Full disclosure: The guilt never fully subsides, but it is lessened by witnessing the growth of your family. Nevertheless, it was challenging; with no nearby familial support and a husband who was mostly at work, my wife took on new stressors that challenged our budding family. I knew I had married a strong, independent, albeit somewhat terrifying woman; however, her ability to not only overcome but also thrive with motherhood surpassed my every expectation.

With our daughter about to turn 2, we have somewhat found our groove (toddlers are somehow more terrifying than newborns?), but like all other aspects of life, there are hills and valleys. There are days when the baby wakes up with a fever and we panic about who can stay home with her, and days where we sit back and take in how lucky we are. The pang of guilt when she repeatedly says "I miss him" while I am at work and the "I love you" when I get home mesh together to create this wonderful and challenging experience. I would not give it up for the world; after all, fatherhood is the best job I have ever had.

Pearls
- Have an open discussion with your partner about your mutual goals as his/her support throughout your journey is key.
- Communicate with your colleagues/residency program and plan ahead of time.
- Carry your share of duties in residency. Others should not pay the price for your life choices.
- Time management is key. Involve your kids in your errands (picking up mail, grocery) to make up for lost times.
- Quality over quantity: make the most of the limited time you have with your family, be present.
- Try to leave work at the door which is not always possible with our jobs, but do it when you can.

Chapter 23
Parental Leave

Kate Watson

Parental Leave

Both men and women receive protection under the 1993 Family Medical Leave Act (FMLA) to take up to 12 weeks of unpaid leave following the birth or adoption of a child [1]. The duration of parental leave taken by surgical residents, however, is most limited by the American Board of Surgery (ABS), which requires 48 weeks of full-time clinical activity per year. Since 2021, the ABS has adopted a new, more flexible policy allowing surgical trainees to take an additional 4 weeks from clinical training for significant life events, including welcoming a new child to the family [2]. This additional leave may be applied to the first 3 years of training and is also available once in the final 2 years of training.

Planning for Parental Leave

Planning for parental leave will vary based on your program. While deciding to make a pregnancy public is different for everyone, the sooner you feel comfortable sharing your need for time away for parental leave, the better. This will allow your program to make plans for coverage for you while you are away. Regardless of the plans, remember that babies do not always come when they are supposed to. Everyone will need to be flexible if your baby comes either before or after expected. Obviously, if your baby comes early, your clinical responsibilities will need to be covered earlier, and your program should develop a contingency plan for if this is the case. However, if your delivery is delayed, make sure to talk with your program

K. Watson (✉)
Oregon Health and Science University, Portland, OR, USA

© The Author(s), under exclusive license to Springer Nature Switzerland AG 2023
A. Ratnasekera et al. (eds.), *General Surgery Residency Survival Guide*, https://doi.org/10.1007/978-3-031-25617-2_23

about what you would want regarding the start date of your leave, as some people may still want to start their leave on the scheduled day, while others may want that time saved for after the delivery of their child.

Maintaining Your Income

Many employers will offer paid leave for a portion of this time, though you will need to check your institutional policies and your employment contract. It may be necessary to use a combination of medical leave, sick leave, vacation, and short-term disability to ensure that your income is maintained. Also pay attention to the percentage of coverage you have with your short-term disability plan, as not all plans cover your salary at 100%. Reviewing your personal plan for leave with your employment benefits or human resources department will help make sure that the logistics surrounding your medical leave goes smoothly.

Once your leave starts, use the time to bond with your child and learn how to be a new parent. Even if it is not your first child, each new addition to the family will change your routine and dynamics. Your family will decide what works best for division of labor and time while you are home. Talk with your partner about how you are going to balance parenting when you go back to work as well. Make sure to be realistic about what your time limitations are going to be once you return to clinical rotations and what remains a challenging and time-consuming occupation.

Preparing to Pump

If you are a woman planning to breastfeed, pumping at work will be one of the challenges you will have to face. Before you go back to work, start planning how you will make pumping at the hospital work, and review the checklist for Breastfeeding at Work and obtain equipment you will need. Speak with co-residents who have also breastfed, and if they do not exist within your own program, find those who have made it work from other programs to learn about institutional resources. Even if you have talked with others before, the last week or so of your leave is a good time to reach out again as you may have more specific questions. Also, if you are planning to use a wearable pump (such as an Elvie, Willow, or similar), once your milk supply is in at home, as you are getting ready to go back to work is a good time to practice with this type of pump.

	Checklist for Breastfeeding at Work
Logistics	
☐	Identify lactation rooms near your workrooms, clinics, and ORs.
☐	Identify fridge locations (if not included with lactation rooms).
☐	Obtain a locker if you do not already have one.
☐	Reach out to other residents who have breastfed for advice.

	Checklist for Breastfeeding at Work
Equipment	
☐	Bag for bringing your pump equipment and supplies each day
☐	Cooler that will fit multiple milk bags and needed snacks
☐	Breast pump
☐	Extra pump parts (tubing, nipple shields, bottles to pump into, or adapters to connect pump bags) to keep at work
☐	Adapters and disposables for if you have access to a hospital-grade breast pump at work
☐	Hand sanitizer/sanitation wipes
☐	Snacks and water
☐	Pens/markers to label milk
☐	Bags for milk if you choose to transfer to storage bags
☐	Backup pump (if possible) or manual pump

Personal Insights

Every single parent I have spoken with has had a unique experience leading up to and following their birth of their child. As a female general surgery resident, my spouse and I knew that he was going to be responsible for a large portion of the parenting responsibilities once I went back to work. Also, as my son was born too small to latch, breastfeeding was logistically (and emotionally) challenging. This meant that while I pumped, my husband was often feeding the baby and doing many of the direct "parenting" responsibilities. I was exhausted during leave and needed every day I had. I was able to take just over 5 weeks of leave given ABS requirements and my decisions regarding vacations and conferences. The week I went back to work was the first week that my milk supply had come in reliably, though I could not deviate from pumping every 3–4 h to maintain it around the clock. I had a friend whose child was 12 min younger than mine, and she had ample supply the entire time, and their division of labor was entirely different than ours, especially as she was breastfeeding entirely, making the childcare and milk production more in sync. I relied heavily on the experiences of my co-residents who had already had children. I did spend the last week of my leave making sure that I knew how to use my Elvie wearable pump which turned out to be a lifesaver when I went back to work, ordered the disposable parts for the Symphony breast pumps which were provided at some of the lactation rooms at work, and got a bag and cooler which allowed me to bring my own pump from home and store the milk. I found that bringing snacks was key—some of the best advice I got was that I could get either lunch or pump—and so I kept food available at all times with the pump equipment. Finally, for me, it made the most sense to pump directly into the milk storage bags to reduce the wasted time transferring milk from containers to bags, so I used the Kiinde system which hooks directly to most of the pump with provided adapters, though we did have some reservations about using so many plastic bags.

Pearls
- Family leave is a legal right protected by the Family Medical Leave Act (FMLA).
- The amount of time taken by surgical residents for the FMLA is generally limited by the American Board of Surgery requirements, which mandate 48 weeks of full-time clinical activity per year, with an additional 4 weeks allowed for significant life events such as welcoming a new child.
- Communicate as early as you are comfortable with your employer to help plan for clinical coverage and also so you can determine how to use your vacation, sick time, and short-term disability as needed to maintain your income.
- If you are a woman planning to breastfeed, make sure to plan early and discuss with other residents and faculty regarding what helped them succeed with breastfeeding while working in your hospital system.

References

1. Congress. Family and medical leave act of 1993. Washington, DC: Congress; 1993.
2. Maloney A. ABS announces more flexible family leave policy for general and vascular surgery trainees. Philadelphia, PA: American Board of Surgery; 2021.

Chapter 24
How to Be There (or Not) for Holidays and Occasions

Johanna Lou

When I was doing a sub-internship as a fourth-year medical student, I remember one particularly busy Friday afternoon. My resident's cell phone had been ringing off the hook with consult after consult. I knew she had a friend's rehearsal dinner that evening and the wedding the next day. As the clock ticked closer to 5 PM sign-out, the rest of the hospital had clearly not understood that she had an important social obligation. I could see the internal struggle as she juggled the onslaught of work. When we got a call for a cold leg late in the afternoon, a true surgical emergency, the phone call she made immediately after the attending and the OR was to her friend, telling her that she was not going to make it that night.

She missed the rehearsal dinner, but on Monday, we were scrolling through pictures on her phone of the wedding. When you become a surgical resident, or any resident for that matter, life around you goes on. One major transition from medical school to residency is the lack of control in your scheduling. While this may improve as you progress in your training, the contrast between the fourth year of medical school and the intern year is jarring. The switch from having nearly every holiday off for the academic year to having no guaranteed holidays requires a change in mindset.

Birthdays, weddings, holidays, and family reunions—they will all still happen. While you may not be able to make all of them, you will still have time off and you will still have the opportunity to be present. It becomes challenging when other important figures in your life, especially those unfamiliar with the rigorous hours of the residency, find it difficult to understand why you are not able to attend every single event. In looking at the experiences of myself and my co-residents, there are a few common themes towards approaching the reality that you will have to learn to prioritize events in your life.

J. Lou (✉)
Cooper University Hospital, Camden, NJ, USA
e-mail: lou-johanna@cooperhealth.edu

A. Ratnasekera et al. (eds.), *General Surgery Residency Survival Guide*,
https://doi.org/10.1007/978-3-031-25617-2_24

Set Expectations

Before starting the intern year, take the space to have a direct conversation with those you care about most regarding the time requirements of your new job. Even several years into residency, I am still greeted with surprise every time I tell my parents that I am working on a holiday. The disappointment or sadness that comes with telling your family you probably cannot make it to Thanksgiving dinner can be mitigated by giving several months of notice. It is also worth mentioning that a surprise visit is almost always more pleasant than a surprise absence.

Take a moment to reflect on what holidays and occasions mean the most to you and your loved ones. Whether picking it means prioritizing a beloved grandmother's 90th birthday over spending Memorial Day Weekend at your annual family barbeque, your family will appreciate being mentally prepared months in advance. Having a frank discussion earlier rather than later can help you prioritize events and figure out the holidays and events in which you want to partake.

Plan Ahead and Communicate Often

Building off the previous point, many programs will pick their vacation schedule at the beginning of every academic year. Our program picks vacations by seniority but allows flexibility for big occasions, such as weddings and trips to visit family abroad. By talking with your family early and communicating with your chief residents and program leadership, you are maximizing your chances of being present for the events that mean the most.

Even the best laid plans go awry, and unfortunately, we are in a field where emergencies happen. If there is even a suspicion that you may need to cancel a plan, give your hosts the courtesy of advance warning. For example, if you are on trauma in the summer when things can be particularly busy at a moment's notice, any RSVP should be accompanied with a large disclaimer that you might need to cancel at the last minute.

Alternative Ways to Celebrate

While missing a holiday can be disappointing, this does not mean that you cannot celebrate. One of the perks of a surgical residency is how closely you work with your co-residents and how many of them become a surrogate family. During my intern year, one of our chief residents hosted a Thanksgiving dinner for any residents who were unable to be with their family. Similarly, another resident who grew up nearby invited several of the residents over her childhood home to celebrate Christmas.

Having flexibility around major events also means that you can still celebrate with your family. During my intern year, I worked on the weekends closest to my father's 70th birthday party. Even though he was disappointed that I missed the formal celebration, I coordinated with my mother to surprise him later in the month. Similarly, for my first 2 years, I was scheduled to be on night float on the day of my wedding anniversary. We ended up making plans for the weekend, when I had off. Even if your schedule does not allow you to celebrate as you would ideally, there are always alternative options.

Celebrate with Your Patients

One of my favorite holidays to work is Christmas. During the intern year when I worked on Christmas, my senior resident and I rounded on a patient with esophageal cancer nearing hospice, and he said that he would always buy his wife a poinsettia plant for Christmas. When our team went down to the cafeteria, we saw some poinsettia centerpieces and were able to purchase one for our patient. When we walked in to do his complex dressing change later in the day, his usual disgruntled grunt when he saw the supplies was followed by a long silence and a quiet "thank you" when he saw the poinsettia.

Oftentimes, a hospitalization over a holiday is unplanned and you will be one of the people who your patients spend their holidays with. I once had an attending sit and watch a quarter of the Super Bowl with one of their patients in the middle of rounds. The day the patient was discharged after a prolonged admission, he asked us to thank our attending for spending that extra time with him. At the end of the day, if you are displeased about working on a holiday, be cognizant that your patients are also spending that day in the hospital. Looking at the situation with a glass-half-full perspective can leave a lasting impact on your patients.

Pearls
- Set expectations with yourself and with your loved ones to establish which life events you want to prioritize.
- Anticipate early and communicate often if you have a commitment that you may not be able to make.
- Embrace nontraditional ways to honor special events, and do not hesitate to celebrate with your patients.

Chapter 25
Finding the Right Home

Johanna Lou

It is easy to feel pressure to participate in the "American Dream" of buying a home as soon as you enter the workforce. Since 1965, homeownership has been over 60%, and at the beginning of 2022, the homeownership rate in the United States was 65% [1]. Before jumping into buying a home, it is important to evaluate personal circumstances, as purchasing a home is not always the best financial decision.

Things to Consider

The first thing to consider is a common piece of home-buying advice called the "5-year rule." This states that you should generally keep a home for at least 5 years before reselling it. Beyond the price of a home itself, there are closing costs, transfer tax fees, and real estate commissions needed in order to buy and sell. This can add up to 7–15% of the cost of the house [2]. Even "all-cash" transactions, where a mortgage loan is not required to purchase the home, can incur some costs and commissions. Lastly, your home will have to appreciate in value to at least the costs of buying and selling just to break even. This is important to consider because a general surgery residency is at least 5 years long, and you might have to move for a fellowship or your first attending position.

If you are interested in keeping the property indefinitely and becoming a landlord when you move, you do not need to worry about the 5-year rule. Or perhaps you are able to purchase a home immediately after medical school and your surgery residency of 5 years is just long enough to recoup those costs even if you have to sell. If neither of these scenarios are applicable to your situation, experts believe that

J. Lou (✉)
Cooper University Hospital, Camden, NJ, USA
e-mail: lou-johanna@cooperhealth.edu

© The Author(s), under exclusive license to Springer Nature   101
Switzerland AG 2023
A. Ratnasekera et al. (eds.), *General Surgery Residency Survival Guide*,
https://doi.org/10.1007/978-3-031-25617-2_25

annual home value appreciation more than 2% per year is considered a "hot market," and you may not be living in a location or market time period where that is the case [2]. All of this is meant to say that it is likely that you will lose money if your plan is to buy a home during residency and sell it upon completion of residency.

Aside from closing costs, you should consider the following future costs when buying a home:

- Property taxes
- Surprise repairs or general maintenance
- Homeowners' association dues (in some cases)
- Insurance
- Utilities that landlords typically cover such as water and heating

A simple way to decide is to take a look at rent versus buy calculators online (NerdWallet has a good one) that consider current interest rates, home prices and rents in your market, as well as typical homeowner costs to determine whether you live in a location where it makes sense to buy a home instead of rent for a few years [3].

Mortgages

Let us say that you have done your research and you have decided that purchasing a home is the right path for you. You may need a mortgage, but you may not have much in savings for a traditional 20% down payment and your debt-to-income ratio may be very high. These are all factors that lenders consider when approving mortgages. Due to substantially higher income potential relative to current salary, residents often qualify for what lenders may call a *physician's mortgage or loan* or a number of other low-moderate-income and first-time home buyer programs.

> "Most physician loans allow you to have a higher-than-normal debt-to-income ratio, which means that you can typically carry more debt, including student-loan debt, which we know a lot of our residents are working through right now," says Laurel Road's Head of Mortgages, Eileen Derks. "You may have a better chance of being approved than you would in a traditional mortgage. So, we're taking all of that into consideration, having confidence and faith that the income trajectory will occur, and the credit quality is there." [4]

Other benefits of physician's loans include bypassing private mortgage insurance (PMI) despite a lower down payment. Most mortgages require private or government mortgage insurance for loans with down payments less than 20%. This is meant to protect the lender should the borrower default on their loan. A physicians' loan is distinctive for not requiring PMI even with a down payment of less than 20%. On large loan amounts, PMI can add hundreds of dollars to the monthly payment [5].

Physicians' loans are not the only types of mortgages that would be a good fit for a resident. Federal and state governments have several programs focused on reducing the barrier to homeownership. There are too many programs to list here and many of them are specific to your home state, but I encourage you to start your research with government resources before moving on to conversations with lenders, brokers, etc. Ensure that your mortgage broker or lender is familiar with programs that can significantly reduce the cost of one of the largest transactions you will ever make.

Here are some good resources to start with:

- *U.S. Department of Housing and Urban Development's Buying a Home Guide*: https://www.hud.gov/topics/buying_a_home
- *First-Time Home Buyer Programs by State (NerdWallet)*: https://www.nerdwallet.com/article/mortgages/first-time-home-buyer-programs-by-state
- *First-Time Home Buyer Programs & Grants*: https://www.fool.com/the-ascent/mortgages/first-time-home-buyer-programs-grants/

Mortgage Pre-approval

Prior to officially starting your home search, you should seek a mortgage pre-approval so that you understand exactly how much you can afford and can move quickly during the offer process. It can be disappointing to find a home you want only to find that the sellers have accepted another offer while you were obtaining your mortgage approval. When accepting an offer, sellers not only look at the offered price but also often take into account the creditworthiness of the borrower. If you have a mortgage pre-approval, chances of your offer getting accepted may be higher.

Most real estate agents will ask you to get one, so they know that you will indeed be able to close the transaction once the offer is accepted. It also helps them get a sense of the price of homes they should help you look for [6]. Obtaining a mortgage pre-approval entails gathering documentation related to identity, income, and assets for all borrowers involved, so start early! It saves you a lot of effort and time later when your offer has been accepted and you are busy doing the many other things involved with home-buying.

Pearls
- Rent vs. buy calculators online can help inform the financial risk/benefit of renting or buying a home.
- When budgeting for your dream home, be aware of additional fees, such as closing costs, transfer tax fees, and real estate commissions that can add up to 7–15% of the cost of the house.
- Physician's mortgages and first-time home-buyer loans can lower the barrier to obtaining a mortgage.
- Prior to officially starting your home search, you should seek a mortgage pre-approval so that you understand exactly how much you can afford and can move quickly during the offer process.

References

1. Homeownership rate in the United States. Federal reserve economic data. https://fred.stlouis-fed.org/series/RHORUSQ156N. Accessed 6 July 2022.
2. Campisi N. Why the 5-year home sale rule still makes sense (most of the time). Bankrate. https://www.bankrate.com/mortgages/5-year-real-estate-rule/. Accessed 6 July 2022.
3. Rent vs buy – what's right for you? NerdWallet. https://www.nerdwallet.com/mortgages/rent-vs-buy-calculator. Accessed 6 July 2022.
4. Murphy B. 4 things to know about buying a home as a resident physician. American Medical Association. https://www.ama-assn.org/residents-students/resident-student-finance/4-things-know-about-buying-home-resident-physician. Accessed 7 July 2022.
5. Lewis H. Physician loans: Flexible mortgage lending for doctors. NerdWallet. https://www.nerdwallet.com/article/mortgages/physician-loans-flexible-mortgage-lending-for-doctors. Accessed 7 July 2022.
6. Sharma S. What's mortgage pre-approval, and how to get one? StemLending. https://www.stemlending.com/mortgage-preapproval/. Accessed 7 July 2022.

Chapter 26
How to Tackle Loan Repayment During Residency

Johanna Lou

In 2020, the Association of American Medical Colleges (AAMC) reported that the median medical school debt was $200,000, not including their undergraduate debt [1]. They also found that the average stipend in a resident or fellow's first year after medical school was $59,279 in 2021 [2]. There are options to defer student loan payments during residency. However, based on the median medical school debt at the federal interest rate, for example, deferring student loans for a 3-year residency would add $31,800 in accrued interest. This would mean a new balance of $231,800, with monthly payments of $2492 on a 10-year payment plan ($342 more than what the monthly payments would be without the deferment) [3]. Thus, it is wise to continue making payments, particularly when income-driven repayment plans are available (Fig. 26.1).

J. Lou (✉)
Cooper University Hospital, Camden, NJ, USA
e-mail: lou-johanna@cooperhealth.edu

Repayment Plans Compared: Which One Works for You?

	Traditional Plans			Income-Driven Plans				
	Standard	Extended	Graduated	Income-Contingent Repayment (ICR)	Income-Based Repayment (IBR) (for those who borrowed before July 1, 2014)	Income-Based Repayment (IBR) (for new borrowers as of July 1, 2014)	Pay As You Earn (PAYE)	Revised Pay As You Earn (REPAYE)
Available in Which Loan Program?	Direct and FFEL	Direct and FFEL	Direct and FFEL	Direct only	Direct and FFEL	Direct only	Direct only	Direct only
What Are the Advantages of This Plan?	May provide the lowest total repayment cost (due to less interest accruing)	Reduced monthly payment, without consolidating	Can offer temporary relief to borrowers expecting an income increase in the near future	Payments may initially be lower than traditional plan payments but will increase as income increases. Capitalized interest cannot exceed 10% of the loan amount that enters the plan. After this, interest accrues but does not capitalize.	Provides affordable payments based on family size and adjusted gross income (AGI) for the household, but there is no limit to interest capitalization	Payments mirror the PAYE payments, but there is no limit to interest capitalization.	May allow for the lowest possible monthly payment. Capitalization cannot exceed 10% of the loan amount that enters the plan. After reaching this limit, interest will accrue but does not capitalize.	May allow for the lowest possible monthly payment. When the monthly payment doesn't cover the interest, you are responsible for only 50% of the accrued and unpaid interest.
How is the Monthly Payment Determined?	Payments calculated equally over the repayment term; payment based on total amount owed	Equal monthly payments stretched over a longer term; payment based on total amount owed	Payments begin lower (interest only in the first 2 years of a 10-year term) and then increase.	Payments are based on the lesser of 20% of your monthly discretionary income or your monthly payment on a plan times a percentage factor based on your income.	Payments are calculated at 15% of your monthly discretionary income and are based on your family size and AGI for the household. The amount is capped at the 10-year Standard payment amount (determined when you enter IBR).	Payments are calculated at 10% of your monthly discretionary income and are based on your family size and AGI for the household. The amount is capped at the 10-year Standard payment amount when you enter IBR.	Payments are calculated at 10% of your monthly discretionary income and are based on your family size and AGI for the household. The amount is capped at the 10-year Standard payment amount (determined when you enter PAYE).	Payments are calculated at 10% of your monthly discretionary income and are based on your family size and AGI for the household. There is no cap on the maximum payment amount.
What is the Repayment Term?	10 years (up to 30 years if consolidated)	25 years	10 years (up to 30 years if consolidated)	Up to 25 years (after which any remaining balance is forgiven but will be taxable)	Up to 25 years (after which any remaining balance is forgiven but will be taxable)	Up to 20 years (after which any remaining balance is forgiven but will be taxable)	Up to 20 years (after which any remaining balance is forgiven but will be taxable)	Up to 25 years for a graduate-level student borrower (after which any remaining balance is forgiven but will be taxable)
What Are the Eligibility Requirements?	Plan available upon request	Must owe more than $30,000 in Direct Loans or FFEL	Available upon request	No initial income eligibility. Payments are based on income and family size.	Must have a Partial Financial Hardship (PFH) to qualify	Must be a new borrower on or after Oct. 1, 2014 and also have a PFH to qualify	Must have a PFH, be a new borrower on or after Oct. 1, 2007, and have a Direct Loan disbursement on or after Oct. 1, 2011. Available only for Direct Loans.	Available only for Direct Loans. There are no additional eligibility requirements.
Does it Qualify for PSLF?	Yes	No	No	Yes	Yes	Yes	Yes	Yes
What Else Should You know about This Plan?	This is the default plan of no other plan is selected. A consolidation loan must be repaid on a 10-year Standard plan (or an income-driven plan) to qualify for PSLF.	This plan will generally cost more than other traditional plans due to the longer repayment term and the resulting increase in interest costs.	The minimum payment is interest only, which can result in higher interest costs compared with the Standard plan.	Income and family size must be verified annually; no cap on the maximum payment amount.	Income and family size must be verified annually. If filing taxes jointly, spouse's income will be considered in eligibility and payments amounts.	Income and family size must be verified annually; payments can be as low as $0/month. If filing taxes jointly, spouse's income will be considered in eligibility and payment amounts.	Income and family size must be verified annually. If filing taxes jointly, spouse's income will be considered in eligibility and payment amounts.	No cap on the maximum payment or on the amount of interest that can capitalize. Income and family size must be verified annually; payments can be as low as $0/month. Spouse's income is always factored into determining the monthly payment.

Fig. 26.1 A comparison of repayment plans [4]

Income-Driven Repayment Plans

Federal student loans offer residents four repayment plans that base a borrower's monthly loan payment on their income. All four plans feature a loan forgiveness benefit. Loan forgiveness occurs after a required 20- or 25-year repayment term is satisfied (dependent upon the repayment plan). A student loan repayment simulator is available on the Federal Student Aid website (studentaid.gov/loan-simulator), which allows you to review scenarios based on your repayment goals. Repayment goals may include paying off loans as quickly as possible or paying the lowest total amount over time.

The four repayment plans include Income-Based Repayment (IBR), Pay As You Earn Repayment (PAYE), Revised Pay As You Earn Repayment (REPAYE), and Income-Contingent Repayment (ICR) [4]. With income-driven repayment plans, the borrower makes a monthly loan payment based on their discretionary income and household size. Two of the plans (IBR and PAYE) also require that the borrower exhibit a partial financial hardship in order to qualify. I encourage you to review the qualification requirements for all four plans on the Federal Student Aid website (studentaid.gov) since they vary based on personal factors, such as your state of residence and the adjusted gross income (AGI) reported on your annual IRS tax filings.

Public Service Loan Forgiveness

If you have federal loans and are employed by a U.S. federal, state, local, or tribal government or not-for-profit organization, you might be eligible for the Public Service Loan Forgiveness (PSLF) Program. In 2020, 76% of community hospitals in the USA were either nonprofit or state, and local government entities and community hospitals make up 85% of all hospitals [5]. Therefore, PSLF is something most medical residents with student loan debt should consider.

Borrowers must make payments to cover 120 separate monthly payments, while working full time (30 h or more per week) for a qualifying employer. After making the required payments on qualifying loans, and meeting the work requirements, the borrower can apply to have their outstanding federal student loan balance forgiven. Borrowers should read the Federal Student Aid website closely, complete annual PSLF paperwork diligently, and track qualifying payments closely to avoid any mistakes that lead to ineligibility. Of note, PSLF is ONLY available for federal Direct Loans. If existing federal student loans did not originate from Direct Loans, they can be converted into a Direct Loan by consolidating [4].

While you may only be able to afford a low monthly payment during residency, once residency training is completed, a physician's salary will increase, and the required monthly student loan payment will also increase. The Federal Student Aid website can help you understand what your monthly payments will be over the years in various income scenarios [6]. Some repayment plans put a cap on what the monthly payment amount can increase to, regardless of income, but not all plans provide this benefit. An income-driven plan paired with meeting PSLF requirements can offer you significant savings on financing your medical education in the long run, as you could experience loan forgiveness in as few as 10 years, including residency and fellowship.

Refinancing Student Loans

I recommend you decide as early as possible whether Public Service Loan Forgiveness will be something you pursue. There are many scenarios where you may not qualify for PSLF, but perhaps you decide you will never complete 10 years of employment at an eligible employer. If that is the case, then you will plan to pay your student loans either in full as soon as possible or at least for 20–25 years prior to being eligible for loan forgiveness through standard federal loan programs. In those scenarios, it may be wise to prioritize saving money on interest by refinancing your loans.

There is no guarantee that a lower interest rate will be available to you. However, if you have a strong credit score, it is possible to find favorable interest rates through loan refinancing with private lenders such as your local bank or other accredited financial institutions. In switching to private lenders, you will lose certain benefits of federal loan programs. It is important to do your research, shop around for the best offer, and weigh the costs and benefits of refinancing (Table 26.1).

Let us compare the costs of paying off $200,000 in federal student loans versus a privately refinanced loan over 20 years using current (July 2022) interest rates. Please note that federal and private interest rates change over time depending on various factors. The Federal Student Aid website lists the most recent graduate or professional borrowing rates at 6.54% for Direct Unsubsidized Loans and 7.54% for Direct PLUS Loans [8]. Let us use the average of these two rates (7.04%) since

Table 26.1 Comparison of the benefits and pitfalls of refinancing federal student loans [7]

Benefits	Pitfalls
You can get a lower interest rate	You are no longer eligible for income-driven repayment
You can pay off your debt faster	You will not qualify for loan forgiveness programs
You can combine multiple loans into one	You are no longer eligible for federal deferment or forbearance
You can relieve your parents of a student loan they may have taken out on your behalf	

Here's what you could save:

You'll save this much each month: You'll save this much in interest:

$343   **$82,426**

How your current loan and refinanced loan compare

Your current loan:

Monthly payment   Total interest paid   Total payments

$1,555.40   **$173,296**   **$373,296**

Your refinanced loan:

Monthly payment   Total interest paid   Total payments

$1,211.96   **$90,870**   **$290,870**

Fig. 26.2 Representative calculation of potential savings after refinancing loans [10]

many students will have a combination of the two loan types. NerdWallet presents a range of private lender rates, depending on your creditworthiness, between 2.69% and 7.99% [9]. In my household, we recently refinanced student loans at a 3.54% interest rate, but let us use a higher 4% for the comparison (Fig. 26.2).

Since private loans typically do not offer income-driven repayment plans, the calculator presents monthly payments for both loans in a standard repayment model. There are many things to consider when making this decision, and this is an example in a vacuum. However, the takeaway is that lower interest rates result in potential savings of tens of thousands of dollars when the loan balance is the average medical student debt burden, and the payback period is potentially 20 years.

Life After Residency

There is no penalty for paying off student loans early, and additional or larger payments will help you pay off the debt faster. But it is also prudent to focus on some additional financial priorities. Some ideas, according to NerdWallet [10], include:

- Establishing an emergency fund to cover 3–6 months of living expenses
- Investing in a retirement fund, at least enough to get your employer's 401(k) match
- Paying down high-interest debt like credit cards

The mean surgeon salary in May 2021 was $294,520, but, if you can continue to live on a resident's budget until your student loans are paid off, you can use the additional income to establish a strong financial foundation.

Pearls
- The Federal Student Aid website has a loan repayment simulator (studentaid. gov/loan-simulator) that can help model a repayment plan given your current financial situation and long-term goals.
- If you have federal Direct Loans and are employed by a U.S. federal, state, local, or tribal government or not-for-profit organization, which many hospitals are, you might be eligible for the Public Service Loan Forgiveness Program.
- It is possible to find favorable interest rates by refinancing your federal loans with private lenders, such as your local bank or other accredited financial institutions.
- Ultimately, there are a lot of factors to consider when determining a strategy for loan repayment, and it is important to balance your day-to-day finances with your future financial health.

References

1. Youngclaus J, Fresne J. Physician education debt and the cost to attend medical school: 2020 Update. Association of American Medical Colleges. 2020 Oct.
2. AAMC survey of resident/fellow stipends and benefits. Association of American Medical Colleges. https://www.aamc.org/data-reports/students-residents/report/aamc-survey-resident/fellow-stipends-and-benefits. Accessed 3 July 2022.
3. Kirkham E. 7 smart strategies for paying off medical school debt. LendingTree. https://studentloanhero.com/featured/pay-off-medical-school-debt/. Accessed 3 July 2022.
4. Income-driven repayment plans and public service loan forgiveness. https://students-residents. aamc.org/financial-aid-resources/income-driven-repayment-plans-and-public-service-loan-forgiveness. Accessed 4 July 2022.
5. Hospitals by ownership type. Kaiser Family Foundation. https://www.kff.org/other/state-indicator/hospitals-by-ownership/. Accessed 5 July 2022.
6. Occupational outlook handbook: physicians and surgeons. U.S. Bureau of Labor Statistics. https://www.bls.gov/ooh/healthcare/physicians-and-surgeons.htm#tab-5.   Accessed   5 July 2022.
7. Tretina K, Hahn A. 8 pros and cons of refinancing federal student loans. Forbes. https://www. forbes.com/advisor/student-loans/refinance-federal-student-loans/. Accessed 5 July 2022.
8. Interest rates and fees for federal student loans. Federal student aid. https://studentaid.gov/understand-aid/types/loans/interest-rates. Accessed 5 July 2022.
9. Clark C. Should I Refinance my student loans? NerdWallet. https://www.nerdwallet.com/article/loans/student-loans/student-loan-refinance-calculator. Accessed 4 July 2022.
10. Nykiel T, Lane R. Paying off medical school debt: 5 strategies for doctors. NerdWallet. https://www.nerdwallet.com/article/loans/student-loans/paying-off-medical-school-debt. Accessed 4 July 2022.

Chapter 27
What We Need in the Workplace

Nishani Hewage

They asked for a baby shower room.

My co-resident is on a committee for designing the new perioperative staff lounge. In a somewhat contentious move, the hospital is combining the OR physician lounge with the OR staff lounge. While that decision was made for us, the designers were otherwise open to hearing our requests for how to use the shared space.

What do we want in the workplace? It is a long list, ranging from the physical (computers that actually work) to the social (supportive colleagues, attendings who care about our well-being).

Let us start with the physical.

There are the basics of the average workplace: computers, desks, bathrooms, a water cooler. Physicians working in the hospital will also need access to food (and lots of coffee) and some call rooms. Surgery residents have additional specific needs, for example operating rooms, a simulation lab, and badge access to the supply room on every unit. A real hot commodity is a Doppler when you are rotating on the vascular surgery service.

A resident-only workspace is critical. Some people even advocate for a separate space for chiefs only. But at the very least, we need a space that is just for us. This is not just where you will run the list with your team, get notes done, and prepare for cases. No, this room is for so much more. This is home base, where the best bonding happens. This is where, in the middle of a 24-h call, you eat pizza while your chief tells everyone crazy stories from years past. This is where you will snap a photo of your co-resident sleeping at a computer and then quietly save it as the desktop background to his or her computer (Fig. 27.1). This is where someday your colleagues might assign a cat from a daily cat calendar to every individual resident and then post each representative cat around the room.

N. Hewage (✉)
Lehigh Valley Health Network, Allentown, PA, USA
e-mail: nishani.hewage@lvhn.org

Fig. 27.1 A comfortable desktop with computer access in the call room

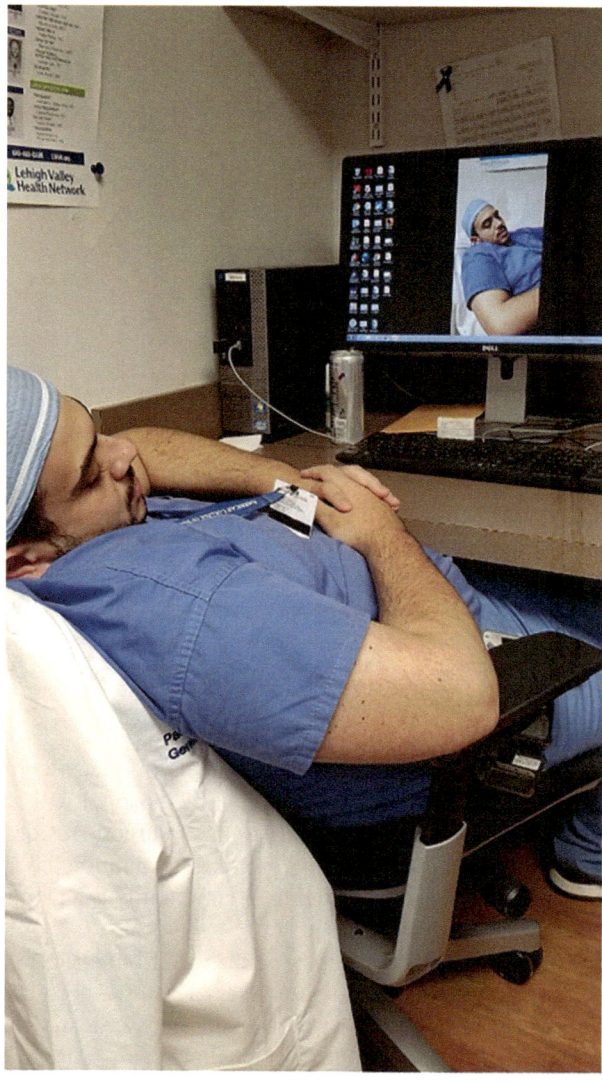

The resident workspace in my hospital is currently within the larger physician staff lounge (for now). This means that the attendings can easily come find us. For us, this is actually nice. Instead of hunting your attending down to force them to make rounds, they will come find you. When they have just accepted five transfers in the span of 5 min, they can pop in to give you a heads-up and look at the CT scans together. Maybe they will drop off leftover food from a department lunch meeting. Or they will come in and grab the Nerf gun someone got in the yearly resident Secret Santa and try to hit an unsuspecting resident at the opposite end of the lounge. Just normal attending things.

See, the key for me is not just having a physical space with computers and a printer, somewhat comfortable chairs, and a couch to rest on (though these are the basic needs for an average surgery resident). More important is to have coworkers and attendings you enjoy working with. Having a supportive and collegial environment will make the worst days a little bit better.

And there will be your "worst" days. Days when your patient has had a terrible complication from something you did to them; days when you meet a patient who has been through something horrific; and days when you must tell a patient and families something devastating that will change their lives forever. All three scenarios may be happening simultaneously. It is the nature of the job. You do not have to be friends with everyone, but at the very least, the compassion we extend to our patients should be similarly directed at our colleagues.

So really, we are not asking for much. What we need in the workplace is simple: good coworkers, a supportive environment …, and, of course, all the basic items for the workplace.

Pearls
- People matter. You will spend more time with your coworkers than anyone else for these 5 years.
- Work hard, and play hard. Do not forget to have fun!
- Eat when you can, sleep when you can … etc.

Chapter 28
Death of a Loved One

Qi Yan Wang

All the training from medical school and surgical residency had prepared me well in taking care of patients, but it is not adequate for handling the death of a loved one. It is an overwhelming experience; whether it occurs expectedly or unexpectedly, we will never be prepared to be ready. Coping the loss can persist years afterwards, and it is a very personalized process. Although there is no hard golden rule, there are some healthy ways for grieving and bereavement:

- *Emotions*
    - You may experience a wide range of emotions, like shock, denial, anger, guilt, regret, sadness, and depression. This is completely normal because you are a human, not a machine!
- *Do not hide*
    - Overcome these emotions by letting them out. You can cry like a baby or scream like a maniac. They will become disruptive or detrimental to life if you hide them for too long.
- *Communication*
    - Have daily conversations with your supporting systems; they could be your chiefs, junior residents, mentors, friends, neighbors, or pets. Your mouth is the door to your mind.

Q. Y. Wang (✉)
Janet Knowles Breast Cancer Center, MD Anderson Cancer Center at Cooper, Camden, NJ, USA

© The Author(s), under exclusive license to Springer Nature Switzerland AG 2023
A. Ratnasekera et al. (eds.), *General Surgery Residency Survival Guide*, https://doi.org/10.1007/978-3-031-25617-2_28

- *Self-care and caring for others*
  - Taking care of yourself is a number one priority. Start with three meals a day and continue routine daily activities. Slow down a minute to watch a sunset, or smell a flower, or walk with a dog, or just take a deep breath.
  - Taking care of others is number two. The loss of a loved one does not stop your role as a mother, a father, a child, a sister, a brother, a friend, a physician, etc. You still have all those duties, responsibilities, obligations, and commitments in life.

- *Memorializing your loved one*
  - Sharing your memory of a loved one is a powerful tool to remind you of his/her existence.

It has been 3 years since my mother passed, but I still remember vividly how terrible that day was. I was a PGY-3 surgical resident covering the service on a Christmas holiday schedule. At about 3 AM, I received a call from my brother "… mom just died …" with a raspy voice. I was in shock, "How it is possible? I just talked to her 2 weeks ago." In FaceTime from thousands of miles away, I saw my mother in her burial gown to come to a realization that my mom had indeed passed!

Feelings of guilt and regret far surpassed my sadness …. My mother was a woman who had a couple of unsuccessful marriages and had worked in a brick factory and washed dishes to raise three kids, one of whom she had not even given birth to herself. Even with her limited middle school-level education, she had taught us to be honest and hardworking people. She never even had a chance to attend our graduations or weddings. Why did she have to be taken? For one and a half years, she lived with me. I was an "excellent" surgical resident but failed to be a qualified daughter. I always thought we would have plenty of time to do something fun next weekend or the next break that never came. Especially since it became necessary for her to rely on a wheelchair for doctor's appointments and she declined in her illness. I became powerless to her saying, "everything tastes like cardboard."

I had figured that it was just a part of disease progression when a patient no longer responds to treatment and hospice care was the final path. I felt sad for the patient's family members when I pronounced their loved ones during my residency training. But I did not really appreciate what this really meant to patients and their loved ones. After 3.5 years of fighting lung cancer, with chemotherapy slowly melting her away, my mother still accepted a new treatment regimen in the hopes of prolonging her life. I felt very frustrated until she told me one day, "your sister only has a couple months left in nursing school, I just want to see her finish if possible." What a humble wish! How could I tell her to stop the treatment? My mother's cancer journey and her subsequent death certainly made me more humble, respectful, and empathetic to patients and their loved ones.

Several months after her death, I immersed myself in my work, pretending to be a happy resident, but I had never felt so empty inside. There was no motivation, hope, or goal. As I approached my fourth year of surgical residency training, I was struggling to decide on the next stage of my life. My mentor said to me one day,

"You lost one mom. Maybe you can save thousands of other people's moms." Being a breast surgeon instantly came to my mind. Yes! This was it! From the cancer diagnosis to the survivorship, I would be there caring for them, being their advocate, and providing hopes for them. What I did not do or what "I should have done" for my mother would be fulfilled.

My mother's death placed me in a dark hole, and for a while, it seemed like I would never see the sunlight. I finally recovered after many months of grief because of so many people supporting me unconditionally. My co-residents, chiefs, attendings, mentors, and my husband. I cried in their arms. They "forced" me to engage in topics and activities other than patient care, to take weekends off, and to eat lunches or dinners with them. But most importantly, it was my mom's love that made me not give up my passion to be a doctor. I continued my path to make her proud as a physician and surgeon counseling many patients and their families through the toughest time of their lives.

There is no easy answer, guide, or solution to deal with the death of a loved one. This was my experience. If you happen to be in an unfortunate situation such as mine, your experience could still be very different from mine. But the "love" will remain the same and become the drive for the rest of your life.

Pearls
- Grieve and bereave by releasing emotions, socializing, caring for oneself and others, and memorializing your loved one.
- The love from the lost ones makes you live today with appreciation and drives you to your future life goals.

Chapter 29
When Your Program Closes

Keshav Kooragayala, Kathryn Eckert, and John Williamson

Introduction

Matching into an accredited surgical residency program is the ultimate goal for medical students who have embarked on the long and arduous path toward becoming a surgeon. For most trainees, the certainty of being locked into a residency program for the duration of their training is associated with tremendous relief and a sense of accomplishment. However, periodically, a hospital will close or lose accreditation, and several residents are faced with this seemingly impossible and uncertain scenario: closure of their surgical training program.

The transition of trainees from resident to "orphan" is unique and uncommon, but unfortunately one that the authors of this chapter have personally experienced. For most surgical residents, the details of the financial and legal aspects dictating residency administration do not have to be considered during training. However, in this chapter, we aim to unveil the legal underpinnings of residency funding and to share practical tips for finding a new residency program. While we hope that no others meet this fate, we endeavor to create a guide for the few trainees who may face a similar situation of hospital or residency program closure in the future.

K. Kooragayala (✉) · J. Williamson
Cooper University Hospital, Camden, NJ, USA
e-mail: kooragayala-keshav@cooperhealth.edu; williamson-john@cooperhealth.edu

K. Eckert
Jersey Shore University Medical Center, Neptune City, NJ, USA

A. Ratnasekera et al. (eds.), *General Surgery Residency Survival Guide*,
https://doi.org/10.1007/978-3-031-25617-2_29

Allocation of Funding for Residency

The funding of individual residency spots is something that most residents have little interest or need to learn. However, in the case of threatened or pending closure of a training program, understanding the process for funding ACGME-accredited residency seats is crucial in allowing a trainee to best face the challenges of finding a position in a new residency program. While the situation in every hospital is unique, funding for residency positions comes from a blend of federally appropriated funds, private donors, hospital funds, and additional state-based funding sources [1].

The federal government is the largest single contributor to GME funding nationally, contributing nearly $16 billion annually (estimated FY 2015), with the bulk of this funding originating from the Centers for Medicare and Medicaid Services (CMS) [2]. This funding is supplemented at the hospital level by private donors, state funding, and individual hospital system contributions. Residency staffing at hospitals is largely determined by the needs of an individual hospital; however, federal funding for these spots is limited by the "cap" established by the Balanced Budget Act of 1997, which froze the number of federally funded training positions at hospitals with established programs [3].

While CMS is the primary stakeholder that funds Graduate Medical Education, it does not regulate the allocation of these funds. The ACGME accredits training programs, allowing them to receive this funding. In training programs operating at or below their "cap," individual programs are responsible for distributing federally received funds to each resident. This per-resident amount (PRA) determines the total dollar amount distributed to each hospital per resident. The sum of money distributed per resident is greater than a trainee's salary, providing supplemental funding for the institution to maintain the overall infrastructure of the training program. In training programs operating above their "cap," institutions supplement federally received money with money from any of the abovenamed sources in order to achieve funding for their full complement of residents. In this situation, the institution often uses its own funding or nonfederal sources of funding to support the infrastructure of its residency program(s).

From the perspective of a trainee whose program is closing, the allocation of residency funding becomes crucial information. While the circumstances of every program closure are different, any and all funding a resident can bring with them to a new program greatly increases their chances of obtaining a new residency training spot. In cases of programs operating at or below their "cap," all federal funding should be transferred with a resident to their new training location. In programs operating above their cap, institutions may be less willing or able to provide nonfederally appropriated funds for residents they are no longer training. While closing programs are encouraged to provide above-cap supplemental funding for all orphaned residents, they are not financially or legally obligated to do so [4].

For example, when examining the closure of Hahnemann University Hospital, residents from surgical specialties with funding were highly desirable to other training programs as adding residents with funding provided the potential for an overall increase in GME's budget. The process of transferring GME funding does theoretically have some uncertainty. When Hahnemann closed, the for-profit parent corporation attempted to claim ACGME-accredited and CMS-funded spots as an asset and sell them at auction. This did not eventually happen as the programs voluntarily resigned accreditation and ACGME reallocated the spots and CMS redistributed funding accordingly. It is unclear if there is no scenario where a hospital and program could try to retain resident funding as a resource even after stopping training.

Additionally, the PRA for each hospital is different and the receiving institutions may have a higher PRA for their own residents in comparison with those they are receiving. This funding discrepancy may leave a gap in the funding of an orphaned resident that will often need to be covered by the new institution. While the entire funding process for residents is beyond the scope of this text, the purpose of this discussion is to highlight the complexity of factors underlying the decision-making process of programs taking on newly orphaned residents.

What to Do in the Immediate Aftermath of Closure

In situations of either an impending closure or a closure that occurs suddenly, the most important first step for residents is to recognize that there is only one stakeholder who truly is invested in their success: themselves. In an ideal situation, the resident's current program director, administrative staff, and teaching faculty are similarly invested in finding a new training spot for their displaced residents. However, due to the varied reasons for program closures, this is not always the case. Faculty and administrative staff are often under pressure to find new jobs themselves, and many have other trainees in different disciplines that are similarly in a difficult situation.

There are a few critical steps that we believe orphaned surgical residents should take in the immediate aftermath of a program closure to best prepare themselves for finding a new training position:

1. *Prepare electronic records of residency application and current credentialing.*

There are significant administrative challenges that are associated with a program closure, and it is important that you have a personal record of your initial ERAS application, an updated curriculum vitae, and an updated ACGME case log record. This last point is of utmost importance, as there is a chance that the electronic case log system may lock out while you are searching for a new program.

2. *Contact the GME office for a description of their role in the process.*

There will be an avalanche of misinformation and conflicting guidance on how to approach the process of finding a new training program. Accordingly, residents should work together to request a written statement regarding the role the GME department will have in assisting trainees as they find new positions. GME will often provide conflicting statements regarding their role in finding new training positions for residents, so obtaining a written statement about GME's plan for facilitating residents' contact with new programs is critical. If GME pledges to make contact for residents at new programs on their behalf, residents should ensure that this process happens swiftly and is well organized. In situations where GME offices are unable to efficiently contact new programs or residents perceive the GME office to be a hindrance to the process, residents should feel empowered to contact potential programs on their own.

3. *Contact the ACGME and local surgical societies.*

While the local GME and hospital administration are important, residents should also reach out to the ACGME and local surgical societies with the assistance of their training faculty. While the ACGME may not be helpful to individual residents, they may be able to provide guidance to local and distant residency programs on the logistical aspects of transferring residents to new positions. They have a national presence allowing them to inform potential residency programs about orphaned residents that they otherwise may not be aware of. In addition, if a program would like to take on a new trainee beyond their ACGME-approved number of positions, the program may need to appeal to ACGME for a temporary increase in their complement of residents in order to accommodate the orphaned resident in their program. Similarly, contacting the local and national surgical societies with the help of faculty may alert other residency programs of the orphaned trainees.

Above all, an orphaned trainee must remember that they are their best and greatest advocate in the process of finding a new training position. They should be prepared to humbly reach out to any contacts they have in the surgical world, and program directors at places they are interested in, to secure themselves a new position. At the same time, they should remember that as residency training funding is severely limited, and surgical subspecialty residents often do significant labor for a hospital further increasing their value, they do have strength in their position. Many Hahnemann residents did end up transferring to programs that they felt were more prestigious and had more resources for training than our original program. Orphaned residents should beware of programs that try to lock them in for transfer quickly and work with a mentor to make sure that once their funding is secured, they are able to transfer to the best possible program for them.

What to Do If You Do Not Find a Spot

While the goal is for every orphaned resident to find a new permanent training location, the reality is that this may not be possible. It is the experience of these authors that with persistence and open horizons, most residents should be able to find a new training location. It is possible, however, that this may not be the case for all involved.

Due to the challenges associated with finding a new position, residents should be prepared to do whatever is necessary to continue their surgical training including relocation, repeating a year of training, or completing a remediation program. Ideally, a candidate would be able to continue training in a geographically convenient location in a positive or consecutive year; however, this may not always be possible depending on the circumstances of a program's closure.

One group that had difficulty finding new programs were residents just beginning their chief year. They brought only 1 year of additional funding with them, and most programs prefer chief residents that know their program's preferences and policies well. In our experience, many of these rising chief residents found success working with the hospitals where they were already matched, or interviewing, for fellowship.

If these measures fail, orphaned surgical residents who remain without a training position may consider taking an unplanned research year or search out positions in other, less competitive, specialties.

The Impact of Residency Closure on Fellowship and Job Prospects

For orphaned residents who can find positions at new surgical training programs in successive years, fellowship and job prospects should not be greatly affected. In fact, residents who can thrive after closure of their initial training program demonstrate resilience that may be viewed favorably during future applications for fellowship or permanent jobs.

As only a few years have passed and we have no controls, we cannot comment objectively on this. However, it has been our observation that all our fellow orphans have been matching as well as we had hoped prior to the program's closure.

Closure of a surgical residency program should never be in the 5–7-year plan of a medical student who has just matched in the surgical training program of their choice. However, if faced with the reality of a program closure, orphaned residents can employ the guidelines above to empower themselves on their journey toward finding a new program at which to complete their surgical training.

Pearls
- An understanding of residency funding processes can be helpful to consider when a program closes.
- In the setting of a program closure, it is critical to collect a record of your residency experience including case logs and credentialing information.
- Contacting academic societies may be helpful to find available programs and increase visibility of your program closure.
- Be prepared to reach out to any previous mentors and colleagues for assistance during this process.
- Ultimately, transitioning to a new residency likely will not affect your fellowship and career goals.

References

1. Pontell ME, Drolet BC. Orphaned trainees: a vulnerable population in an inequitable system. J Surg Educ. 2022;79(1):17–9.
2. He K, Whang E, Kristo G. Graduate medical education funding mechanisms, challenges, and solutions: a narrative review. Am J Surg. 2021;221(1):65–71.
3. Butkus R, Lane S, Steinmann AF, Caverzagie KJ, Tape TG, Hingle ST, et al. Financing U.S. graduate medical education: a policy position paper of the alliance for academic internal medicine and the American College of Physicians. Ann Intern Med. 2016;165(2):134–7.
4. Aizenberg DJ, Logio LS. The graduate medical education (GME) gold rush: GME slots and funding as a financial asset. Acad Med. 2020;95(4):503–5.

Part IV
Leadership/Ethics

Chapter 30
Leadership

Hakan Orbay and Toba Bolaji

Introduction

"A team is a small number of people with complementary skills who are committed to a common purpose, performance goals, and approach for which they hold themselves mutually accountable" [1]. In this sense, residents and other healthcare personnel working together in a hospital constitute a team. Effective teams need individuals with different skill sets (i.e., junior and senior residents, nurses, surgical technologists) and a designated leader. Surgeons are usually the leaders of teams within the healthcare system [2].

The definition of a good surgeon has evolved over the years. A thirteenth-century French Army surgeon, Henri de Mondeville, described a good surgeon as follows: "The most important requirement for a good surgeon is a strong stomach and ability to cut like an executioner." Later, Sir William Osler introduced the term "triple-threat clinician" [3]. He described the ideal academic surgeon as the one who 1. performed original primary research, 2. trained medical students and residents, and 3. provided high-quality clinical care. For years, these criteria were used by academic facilities to hire physicians. There was no emphasis on leadership skills and nontechnical skills of a surgeon [3]. However, with the recent changes in the culture and environment of our profession, becoming a successful academic surgeon requires more than being a "triple-threat clinician." Surgeons need technical skills and a steady hand and are expected to have the knowledge, skills, and attitudes to achieve the established goals of our teams [2–4].

H. Orbay (✉)
Crozer Chester Medical Center, Upland, PA, USA
e-mail: orbayh@upmc.edu

T. Bolaji
ChristianaCare Health System, Newark, DE, USA
e-mail: oloruntoba.o.bolaji@christianacare.org

A. Ratnasekera et al. (eds.), *General Surgery Residency Survival Guide*,
https://doi.org/10.1007/978-3-031-25617-2_30

127

Surgery is increasingly multidisciplinary, and the traditional, authoritarian leadership style of the stereotypical surgeon is no longer tolerated and is considered to be unprofessional. As a response to this increasing demand and gap in the leadership training of surgical residents, national organizations have developed leadership training programs. The "Leadership Skills Training Program for Chief Residents" was developed by the Accreditation Council for Graduate Medical Education (ACGME) [5] (Fig. 30.1), and the "Residents as Teachers and Leaders (RTAL)" course was developed by the American College of Surgeons (ACS) specifically for senior residents in surgical specialties [6]. Leadership has also been recognized as a core professional competency for all doctors, and a separate skill domain within the nontechnical skills of surgeons (NOTSS) program [7]. The goal is to develop a non-authoritarian leadership style to lead and promote team members and to give the courage to speak up against inappropriate leadership behaviors [8].

Many surgical trainees lack fundamental understanding of the complexity of leadership. It is a common misconception to think of leadership merely as a process of telling the other team members what to do [9]. However, as surgeons, our behaviors and interpersonal relations determine the work environment, team dynamics, satisfaction, and overall performance of the team [10]. Introducing leadership skills early in the protected environment of residency paves the road for a successful career [11]. So, what determines a good leader in this era?

A good leader is one with self-awareness, self-management, and empathy to the expectations and the problems of other team members. The leader of a team should model the way, inspire a shared vision, challenge the process, and enable and encourage the others to act (Table 30.1) [11–13]. There are different leadership styles (Table 30.2). Even though one leadership style might not be the best for every situation, the one with the highest rate of appreciation from the other team member is "*visionary leadership*" followed by "*coaching-style leadership*" [14]. Leadership is a dynamic concept; it may be necessary to switch between leadership styles

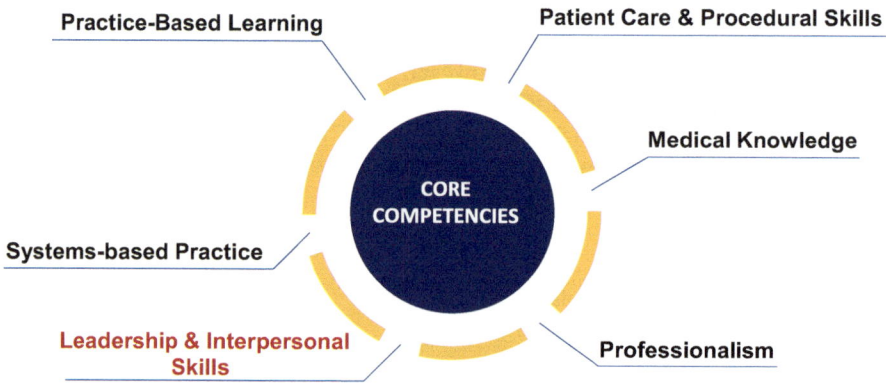

Fig. 30.1 Six core competencies defined by the Accreditation Council for Graduate Medical Education (ACGME) and the American Board of Medical Specialties (ABMS). Adapted from the Royal Australasian College of Surgeons [7]

Table 30.1 Behavioral patterns associated with good leadership. Adapted from the Royal Australasian College of Surgeons

- Identifies when to lead, manage, or take direction as required
- Adjusts leadership style and mentoring according to the most appropriate method for the recipient
- Is willing to take direction from colleagues when advised to
- Encourages trainees and junior staff to lead a situation with backup support as needed
- Leads to inspire others
- Acts as a role model to others in both technical and nontechnical areas of surgery
- Remains calm under pressure, working methodically towards effective resolutions of difficult situations
- Resolves team conflicts quickly and appropriately
- Seeks assistance when unexpected technical problems arise
- Speaks up about patient safety issues
- Sets and maintains standards
- Introduces self to new or unfamiliar members of the surgical or practice team
- Clearly follows hospital, operating theatre, ward and practice protocols
- Requires all team members to observe standards
- Seeks opportunities to participate in local health district quality and standards advisory committees
- Supports others
- Offers understanding and flexibility to colleagues who are experiencing difficulties inside or outside the workplace
- Organizes operating lists to ensure that there is time for trainees and junior staff to have supervised hands-on experience
- Encourages and facilitates briefing and debriefing procedures involving the entire team
- Provides supportive feedback to team members including on areas that need improvement

Table 30.2 Leadership styles

Visionary	These leaders are inspirational and also emotionally intelligent. They encourage their team to "innovate, experiment, and take calculated risks"
Coaching	This type of leader focuses on the professional development of individuals, helping them to improve their skill set and accomplish the goals of the organization
Affiliative	This style focuses on nurturing teamwork and connecting people
Democratic	This style relies on the consensus and collective wisdom of a group of people
Pacesetting	This leader is driven by results, constantly searching for ways to do things better and faster
Commanding	The leader focuses on giving clear directions

depending on the complexity of each situation. For example, in a crisis situation, a direct, assertive, and driven leadership style may be the most effective, but will most likely fail if used every day during routine day-to-day situations, such as routine morning rounds or operations [9].

As surgeons, our competence and performance are closely related to the trust that we receive from other team members; hence, leaders, while providing direction to the team, should demonstrate high standards of clinical practice and care [2]. Nothing will dampen motivation, initiative, and sense of ownership more than an inconsistent leader. As leaders, always hold yourself to a higher standard and lead by example. Take ownership of your team, accept blame when the team falls short, and acknowledge the contribution of the other team members to the success of the team [12]. Establish a good rapport with the team members, and check in and offer support when someone seems to be struggling [12].

Delegation is an important aspect of leadership. Picking the right person to manage a problem can grow both the "leader" and the "doer." However, a leader can delegate tasks but not the responsibility. Leaders should also learn to become effective followers when the problem at hand is within the expertise of another team member. Failure to do so creates dysfunctional teams to the detriment of patient care [2].

Leading a surgical team has unique challenges. The members of a surgical team are well-educated and highly trained professionals. Such people are keen on their autonomy, and they prefer to be consulted. They need to be engaged and kept involved and must have some "buy-in" to the task at hand. They value freedom and flexibility while performing the tasks delegated to them [2]. Therefore, physicians should involve their colleagues in the decision-making process and avoid micromanaging the members of the team.

Pearls
- Society is a dynamic structure that continuously evolves. Behaviors that were largely accepted in the past have become outdated and unpopular within time. As surgeons, it is our responsibility to be current with the new concepts and guidelines in our profession.
- Adaptability is crucial for survival, and the surgeons who cannot adapt to new trends and insist on keeping the old habits are bound for failure. It is not only a steady hand and a strong will that define a good surgeon, but modern surgeons are expected to excel in social skills.
- Practicing modern leadership skills early during residency will pave the road for a successful career.

References

1. Katzenbach JR, Smith DK. The wisdom of teams: creating the high-performance organization. Boston, MA: Harvard Business Press; 1993.
2. Watters DA, Smith K, Tobin S, Beasley SW. Follow the leader: followership and its relevance for surgeons. ANZ J Surg. 2019;89(5):589–93.
3. Morris MC, Baker JE, Edwards MJ. Surgeons, scholars, and leaders symposium: a 5-year experience. Am Surg. 2019;85(12):1327–33.
4. Hill DA MD, Jimenez JC, Cohn SM, Price MR. How to be a leader: a course for residents. Cureus. 2018;10(7):e3067.
5. Accreditation Council for Graduate Medical Education. Improving physician well-being RMiMC, Illinois, United States. Available at: https://www.acgme.org/what-we-do/initiatives/physician-well-being.

6. American College of Surgeons. Residents as Teachers and leaders, Illinois, United States. Available at: https://www.facs.org/education/division-ofeducation/courses/residents-as-teachers.
7. Updated surgical competence and performance guide. Royal Australasian College of Surgeons, 2020. https://www.surgeons.org/-/media/Project/RACS/surgeons-org/files/Louise-Pfrunder/Surgical-Competence-and-Performance-Framework_V16.pdf?rev=120ec964eb9e4c26a1f266 eba17eaf79&hash=BA49820B4620667CA9F007C72856E346.
8. Flin R, Yule S, Paterson-Brown S, Rowley D, Maran N. The non-technical skills for surgeons (NOTSS) system handbook. Aberdeen: University of Aberdeen and Royal College of Surgeons of Edinburgh; 2006.
9. Barnes T, Rennie SC. Leadership and surgical training part 2: training toolkit for leadership development during surgical training. ANZ J Surg. 2021;91(6):1075–82.
10. Leach LS, Myrtle RC, Weaver FA. Surgical teams: role perspectives and role dynamics in the operating room. Health Serv Manag Res. 2011;24(2):81–90.
11. Lases LS, Arah OA, Busch OR, Heineman MJ, Lombarts KM. Learning climate positively influences residents' work-related well-being. Adv Health Sci Educ. 2018;5:1–4.
12. Kostka R, Fleshman JW. Leadership in surgical residency. Clin Colon Rectal Surg. 2020;33(4):221–4. https://doi.org/10.1055/s-0040-1709438. Epub 2020 Jul 1
13. Kouzes J, Posner B. The leadership challenge. How to make extraordinary things happen in organizations. 5th ed. San Francisco, CA: Jossey-Bass; 2012.
14. Goleman D, Boyatzis R, McKee A. Primal leadership: unleashing the power of emotional intelligence. Boston, MA: Harvard Business Press; 2013.

Chapter 31
Fundamentals of Professionalism

Nosayaba Enofe and Hakan Orbay

Introduction

Healthcare professionalism is a core competency for medical trainees and practicing physicians [1, 2]. The Association of American Medical Colleges (AAMC) published the *Assessment of Professionalism Project* in 1995, with examples of behaviors to guide defining professionalism in medicine for trainees, students, and practicing physicians [1]. Since then, professionalism curricula for medical trainees have multiplied and over the past decades have begun to underscore the importance of humanistic and ethical reflections rather than behavioral observations alone [1]. In 1999, the Accreditation Council for Graduate Medical Education (ACGME) identified professionalism as one of Six Core Competencies for resident training and evaluation [2, 3]. Residents must demonstrate the ability to acquire and showcase this unique skill set as part of the requirements for successful completion of residency training and certification to practice as a physician or surgeon. In this chapter, we explore the concept of professionalism and discuss the subcompetencies that make up the ACGME professionalism Core Competency, thus providing a framework for residents to become proficient in this attribute.

Professionalism is largely the behavioral characteristic of a professional summarized by one's skills, competency, courtesy, and ethics. Simply put, it is the ability to take one's work seriously and master the craft with ethical obligations, while at the same time showing sensitivity and respect to self and everyone encountered amid the practice of a profession [4, 5]. It is underpinned by the professional identity which undergoes a process of well-documented formation in medicine [1, 6]. Medical professional identity formation (PIF) experiences its greatest transformation during the transition from the medical student to the resident and the

N. Enofe (✉) · H. Orbay
Crozer Chester Medical Center, Upland, PA, USA
e-mail: Nosayaba.enofe@fccc.edu

© The Author(s), under exclusive license to Springer Nature Switzerland AG 2023
A. Ratnasekera et al. (eds.), *General Surgery Residency Survival Guide*,
https://doi.org/10.1007/978-3-031-25617-2_31

resident to the practicing physician [1]. While formal professionalism education curriculum exists at medical schools, residents' exposure to professionalism is largely nonstructured education and role modeling. The ACGME therefore outlines and describes a set of subcompetencies to illustrate the Core Competency of medical professionalism by which residents are longitudinally educated, evaluated, and expected to successfully master prior to completion of training [2, 3]. Programs assess this core competency using multisource feedback including patient surveys and direct observation [3, 7].

A review of the medical professionalism literature reveals that altruism, integrity, excellence, compassion, continuous improvement, and working in partnership are expressions used to describe the values of medical professionalism [8, 9]. Residents are expected to act ethically and in the best interest of the patient at all times, placing the needs of others above theirs; demonstrate a commitment to professional and self-development, and pursuit of knowledge and excellence; display reliability and empathy; be sensitive to diverse cultural backgrounds and views; interact in a respectful and dignifying manner with patients, family members, colleagues, and all individuals in the workplace; and take responsibility for how their time is planned and spent working within the ACGME duty hour restriction [2, 7]. Although residents are expected to be altruistic, the physical and mental health of the resident should remain paramount, and residents should be empowered to seek and maintain good health as part of the concept of professionalism. Burnout, substance use, mental illness, and suicides are leading causes of physician health deterioration, and therefore, programs must first equip residents with the tools required to maintain their mental and physical heath and residents should in turn demonstrate a commitment to self-care and preservation [8].

Three subcompetencies form the cornerstone of graduate medical education (GME) professionalism assessment: professional behavior and ethical principles, accountability and conscientiousness, and self-awareness and help-seeking [7, 10]. The ACGME further streamlines these subcompetencies to include the following: *(i)* demonstrating professional conduct and accountability—which has to do with punctuality, honesty, integrity, work preparedness, physical presentation, dedication to knowledge, self- and technical improvement, self-awareness, understanding limitations and seeking out counsel, team player, and always maintaining ethical conduct; *(ii)* demonstrating humanism and cultural proficiency—reflects humane behaviors and relationship building, recognizing the self-worth and dignity of others, respectful interactions at all times, privacy and confidentiality, patient advocate, empathy, socioeconomic and cultural sensitivity, and inclusivity; and, finally, *(iii)* maintaining emotional, physical, and mental health, and pursuing continual personal and professional growth—refers to health sustenance and maintenance, healthy lifestyle and choices, commitment to lifelong learning and continuous medical education, desire for self-growth and improvement, frequent conference attendance, seeking out feedbacks, and favorably responding to constructive criticisms [2, 3].

Professionalism in medicine is therefore at the core of what makes a successful medical practitioner. It is the bedrock of all six ACGME core competencies and a continual process of introspective self-growth refining behavior and attitudes. A mastery of this is fundamental to providing quality healthcare. Residents should be taught this concept, preferably in a formal curriculum, and understand the subcompetencies by which programs evaluate medical professionalism.

Pearls
- Learning professionalism early in one's career has huge long-term benefits.
- Spend time learning the ACGME core competencies, and obtain an understanding of how residents are evaluated during residency.

References

1. Reimer D, Russell R, Khallouq BB, Kauffman C, Hernandez C, Cendán J, et al. Pre-clerkship medical students' perceptions of medical professionalism. BMC Med Educ. 2019;19(1):239.
2. NEJM Knowledge+ Team, Drazen JM. Exploring the ACGME Core competencies: professionalism (Part 7 of 7). N Engl J Med. 2017; https://knowledgeplus.nejm.org/blog/acgme-core-competencies-professionalism/. Accessed 22 June 2022
3. Edgar L, McLean S, Hogan SO, Hamstra S, Holmboe ES. The milestones guidebook. Accreditation Council for Graduate Medical Education (ACGME); 2020.
4. Merriam-Webster Dictionary. "Professionalism". In: Merriam-Webster. 2022. https://www.merriam-webster.com/dictionary/professionalism. Accessed 22 June 2022.
5. Dictionary.com. Professionalism. 2022. https://www.dictionary.com/browse/professionalism. Accessed 22 June 2022.
6. Shapiro J, Nixon LL, Wear SE, Doukas DJ. Medical professionalism: what the study of literature can contribute to the conversation. Philos Ethics Humanit Med. 2015;10:10.
7. Frohna JG, Padmore JS. Assessment of professionalism in the graduate medical education environment. J Grad Med Educ. 2021;13(2 Suppl):81–5.
8. The Lancet. Medical professionalism and physician wellbeing. Lancet. 2021;398(10303):817.
9. Rothman DJ, Blumenthal D, Thibault GE. Medical professionalism in an organizational age: challenges and opportunities. Health Aff (Millwood). 2020;39(1):108–14.
10. Edgar L, Roberts S, Holmboe E. Milestones 2.0: a step forward. J Grad Med Educ. 2018;10(3):367–9.

Chapter 32
Art of Delegation

Ryan Gordon

Introduction

One may propose that the "art of delegation" is the task order as delegated by the command or, in this case, the senior resident. That is only partially true; however, the delegation of duties is truly at all levels. This delegation can trickle down to your junior colleagues, medical students, and even oneself. Alas, the demonstration of beautiful execution of the art of delegation must also trickle up to the attending level. At the end of the day, this comes down to understanding of the team's mission and having camaraderie amongst the team, and thereafter delegation at all levels will not just be a concept but a group ethos.

The Junior Resident

In many places, the task assigned to the junior resident is typically at the initial encounters with the patient. An example would be seeing consults, dealing with floor patients, dispositions, and following rounds with the senior or attending. This is a thankless job. Everyone knows this, but it allows for the appreciation of every tier of surgery. The tasks delegated to them are mission essential. But the art of delegation applies to the junior resident as well. As mentioned before, even the intern is now the chief to medical students, who are looking up to the intern.

R. Gordon (✉)
ChristianaCare Health System, Newark, DE, USA
e-mail: ryan.d.gordon@christianacare.org

A. Ratnasekera et al. (eds.), *General Surgery Residency Survival Guide*,
https://doi.org/10.1007/978-3-031-25617-2_32

137

Being in delegated tasks is part of the job. However, not seeing the walls of the OR can make such tasks seem less appealing and can lay a burden on the mind. However, it is the chief resident's job to explain how important everything done at the junior level is mission critical. Seeing a consult and staffing it quickly streamline care. The patient will remember YOU in the emergency room and afterwards on the floor.

The junior resident should learn as much as possible and do as much as possible. It is their opportunity to showcase their efficiency and attention to detail. But the junior can delegate one's own tasks for themselves. One way is to develop a unique shorthand way to take notes. Everyone knows the fishbone diagrams for labs, but this can be done for patients in many ways. Make it for every service. For example, make a "T" on the patient's section of your list. Atop the "T," put the diet; at the bottom left of the "T," put + or − for passing flatus; and at the bottom right of the "T," put + or − for a bowel movement. Now you have literally changed words into a few strokes of the pen, and the information is still there for those bowel obstruction patients. The intern should develop shortcuts to every administrative task possible and allow more time for patient care at bedside or time in the operating room. Your administrative efficiency will be perceived as excellent time management and should allot the opportunity for advanced skills (such as yielding the scalpel, leadership opportunities within the department and residency).

The Senior Resident

Delegating tasks as a senior resident is, for the most part, easy. The senior says "do this" and the junior is expected to execute it. That is how the basics of the dichotomy of task delegation works. Just like a child compared to the parent or the junior enlisted soldier to the commanding officer. This is your task, and it needs to get done. If you have a good team, then it is seamless. If you have a challenging team, make cohesion, an environment of trust, accountability, and opportunity for all to feel the success together. Mission success equates to everyone's victory.

Concept of Fluid Dichotomy

There is dichotomy and order of rank; however, there must exist the ability to be fluid to allow for others to step up as well as leaders to step a rank, or more, lower. This lead-by-example style will allow others to feel that they have opportunities above their PGY to broadcast their leadership/skills and allow the junior residents to see that no task is above the senior resident. Soon, other residents will step up to help the struggling intern, stay late with the senior to do a case, and realize the opportunities for mid-level leadership. Hence, as the senior resident, you may burden yourself with seemingly junior-level tasks at times, but the team will see your commitment to the team and soon they too will extend themselves without seeming like a burden to the team's success. Once the team has this level of fluid dichotomy, the leader will be able to delegate tasks without groans, but more of excitement for the opportunity.

Now to actual delegation for the upper tier resident. The art of delegation should truly be based on the concept of educating the resident (any level) and pushing them to the next level. Yes, the junior residents will have to handle the frontline battle of consults and floor dilemmas. But giving them the opportunity to get into the operating room will give them a taste of what they are working for. In surgery, much like the military, there has to exist hierarchical schemes to create the flow of patient care. With that in mind, senior residents must give the juniors, even interns, the chance to play or see what opportunity lies after the scut work. This will prevent burnout as well as keep them motivated to stay on the attack for the team. Now, there are levels of tasks appropriate for PGY, but I would challenge that chief to push the boundaries on this concept. Taking the consult resident in on any case will motivate them. But what if you asked them to start the case and then you take it over when appropriate? Task them with teaching the medical student to close the wounds, and then you, the senior, breaks scrub. It will put the responsibility and heat on the junior to foster basic leadership and demonstrate knowledge/skills, and make them feel trusted to take command. It is a dual task in challenging teaching for the senior and a ticket to Disneyland for the junior.

Getting a Heavy Load Uphill

Once the team leadership scheme is set, the art of delegation now becomes a much easier task. But what if that is not the case? What if the team does not gel or there is animosity amongst its members? What if the leader is struggling to delegate and motivate? What specifically in the realm of delegation can one do?

Start from the bottom. It is okay to tell the team that there is a lack of cohesion or understanding of what the team is trying to do. Reiterate what everyone's role is and explicitly say it. Now everyone at a bare minimum understands what the expectations are. From there, reattempt to integrate the fluid leadership ideals once the team has demonstrated that their expectations are met. Sometimes, this means thinking outside the box; this can include utilization of less invasive environments for fostering the team. This can be team lunch, team workouts, team happy hour, going to a local event, or having them over for dinner. Attendings are a great source to help with this too. Whatever the leader thinks will allow a less hostile, open environment for banter and fostering human interaction. Again, find things where people can talk about work, laugh, and find inherent camaraderie without the pressure of being on the clock. In time, one will find that the team will just click. Seemingly less attractive tasks for juniors will miraculously be executed fast, thoroughly, and potentially with enthusiasm. The senior will have fulfillment in having a well-oiled machine.

Ultimately, remember that it is the "art" of delegation. New teams may demand different tactics. Residency is not just learning about the "art" of taking care of the patient, but it is also about molding your style of leadership and delegation.

Pearls
- Delegation is a universal at all levels of a surgical career.
- Art of delegation requires one to act by example, give reward, and understand team dynamics.

Chapter 33
"Sticks and Stones … But Words Do Hurt"

Toba Bolaji

Most surgical residents are familiar with the jarring experience of operating with a surgeon with a condescending attitude and a short temper. It is one of those situations where it seems like nothing is going in your favor. As soon as you are handed the scalpel, he/she makes a snide comment about why you are holding it incorrectly. No bite of your stitch is perfect enough. It is never the right angle or the amount of tissue they wanted. As the case continues, you grow more frustrated, but you know reacting will only make the situation worse. It gets to the point where you are more focused on what the attending is going to say next than the case. You are traumatized at the end of the case and question your knowledge and ability.

Residency training is built on an apprenticeship-like model, marked by graduated autonomy and hierarchy. Developed in the early 1900s, graduated autonomy is the cornerstone of the system used to train young physicians. It is this infrastructure that guides the development of medical knowledge and practical skills that are sequential, logical, and safe. Intrinsic to this is a hierarchical system of providers, which often predisposes to a hierarchical culture. Though it is necessary to have a system that allows learning but keeps patients safe, the hierarchical nature of this system has concordantly led to an often psychologically unsafe and toxic culture, one that often allows for a culture of bullying [1]. Frankly, bullying should have no place in the medical environment. In a culture that promotes health and wellness for our patients, that same standard should permeate the interactions amongst providers [2]. Toxic work environments within the medical space have long been propagated by power dynamics that span the differences in age, gender, race, sexual orientation, and disability. Within a profession that has long been primarily occupied by Caucasian cisgender males, the diversity of providers that we continue to now see has come with issues of bullying and microaggressions [3].

T. Bolaji (✉)
ChristianaCare Health System, Newark, DE, USA
e-mail: oloruntoba.o.bolaji@christianacare.org

A. Ratnasekera et al. (eds.), *General Surgery Residency Survival Guide*,
https://doi.org/10.1007/978-3-031-25617-2_33

141

A work environment that allows and enables bullying, discrimination, and the prevalence of microaggressions can negatively impact a person's own health and career. An understated by-product of that is the effect it can have on the workforce at large and its patients. Further, bullying leads to increased turnover, lower attrition of specific demographics, higher incidence of mental health issues, and decreased satisfaction in the job.

Johns Hopkins Medicine defines bullying in the workplace as "unwanted, recurring aggressiveness that causes psychological or physical harm, and creates a psychological power imbalance between the bully and the targets" [4].

As a resident/trainee, dealing with bullying is not easy. The power dynamics intrinsic to the medical environment are not in your favor, and the fear of being ignored, minimized, and even retaliated against is understandable. First, the importance of having a strong support system outside the hospital cannot be overstated. People who know, appreciate, and love you allow you to keep perspective during rigorous training. The value of having a support system to lean on during times when you may feel victimized is priceless. Building support systems within the hospital is equally important. You need mentors that are invested in your wellness and development as a young physician. In times when you are a victim of bullying, your mentors can use their senior position to advocate on your behalf and provide further wisdom on how to deal with difficult situations.

Sometimes, avoidance is a valuable tool to protect your own physical and mental health and overall peace from workplace bullies. Whenever possible, avoid unnecessary contact with individuals who cross those boundaries. Be careful that this avoidance does not come at the expense of patient care. When it does, this is a clear sign that the issue needs to be escalated and dealt with [5].

Microaggressions, defined by Johns Hopkins Medicine, are "verbal, behavioral or environmental indignities, whether intentional or unintentional, that communicate hostile, derogatory or otherwise negative prejudicial slights and insults toward any individual or group, particularly culturally marginalized individuals" [4]. Often dealt with by people within marginalized communities, microaggressions can be hurtful words or actions, not even recognized by the perpetrator. As with bullying, they can have damaging effects to an individual's physical and mental health and contribute to the imposter syndrome and burnout that many, especially marginalized, communities feel in these high-standard, high-pressure environments. Microaggressions need to be taken seriously, because at its core, such comments and actions are disrespectful and are a sign of cultural inequality and inequity [6]. At the individual level, the importance of addressing microaggressions cannot be overstated. Georgetown University School of Medicine has developed a communication guidance tool that coaches medical students and residents on an appropriate approach to dealing with microaggressions. Stop, talk, and roll is a tool that encompasses suggested phrases and approaches in specific circumstances. Stop means to make a mental note of the interaction and judge the appropriateness of addressing the matter in the moment or later. Talk prompts an interjection of this conversation that either addresses or diffuses the interaction. Lastly, roll is the act of finding the proper individuals or systems that can help to review, debrief, and interrogate the situation [3].

At the systemic level, organizations should work to build and cultivate workplaces that promote candid conversations around difficult and nuanced subjects like sexism, racism, and homophobia. The more we can create environments where these issues are talked about, the more aware we are of crossing the boundaries of microaggressions, and hopefully, the less it happens [6].

Bullying and microaggressions are workplace issues that pose a threat to physical and mental health and overall well-being. Surgical education is especially susceptible to issues given its hierarchical culture and the innate level of stress involved in the job [7]. Both should be addressed early at the individual level to mitigate their long-term effect, but more importantly, systems and employers should intentionally build systems that prevent and address these issues as they arise.

Pearls
- Bullying and microaggressions have been a negative by-product of the hierarchical nature of medical and surgical education.
- Bullying should never be tolerated in the healthcare workplace.
- Bullying and microaggressions can have damaging effects to an individual's physical and mental health.
- It is important to have a strong support system both inside and outside of the hospital.
- Avoidance of potential bullying situations should not be happening at the compromise of patient care. This is a clear sign that the issue needs to be escalated.
- Microaggressions are a sign of cultural inequality and inequity.
- Stop, talk, and roll is a communication guidance tool that can be used to handle specific circumstances of microaggressions.
- Organizations should work to build a work environment that promotes honest and empathetic conversations about these issues.

References

1. Samora J. Occurrence of discrimination, bullying, & harassment in the medical profession -- and its importance [online]. Cpb-us-e1.wpmucdn.com. 2022. Available at https://cpb-us-e1.wpmucdn.com/sites.uw.edu/dist/9/4123/files/2019/12/Samora_harassment_3.6.2019.original.1552080639.pdf. Accessed 25 June 2022.
2. Murphy B. Workplace bullying must have absolutely no place in medicine [online]. American Medical Association. 2022. Available at https://www.ama-assn.org/practice-management/physician-health/workplace-bullying-must-have-absolutely-no-place-medicine. Accessed 25 June 2022.
3. Department of Allied Health Sciences. Microaggressions/Micro affirmations | Department of Allied Health Sciences [online]. 2022. Available at https://www.med.unc.edu/ahs/about-us/diversity/jeditoolkit/microaggressions-microaffirmations/. Accessed 25 June 2022.
4. Nitken K. Bullying, microaggression and other terms [online]. Hopkinsmedicine.org. 2022. Available at https://www.hopkinsmedicine.org/news/articles/bullying-microaggression-and-other-terms. Accessed 25 June 2022.

5. Llewellyn A. How to deal with bullies in medicine. 8 Tips for surviving [online]. AdvanceMed. 2022. Available at https://advancemed.com.au/blog/how-to-deal-with-bullies-in-medicine/. Accessed 25 June 2022.
6. Washington E. Recognizing and responding to microaggressions at work [online]. Harvard Business Review. 2022. Available at https://hbr.org/2022/05/recognizing-and-responding-to-microaggressions-at-work. Accessed 25 June 2022.
7. Taylor-Robinson S, De Sousa Lopes P, Zdravkov J, Harrison R. A personal perspective: is bullying still a problem in medicine? Adv Med Educ Pract. 2021;12:141–5.

Chapter 34
Facing Complications

Arielle Brackett

Introduction

Residents will hear many different surgical aphorisms throughout their training. Some of the most common include quips like "Surgery is a contact sport," "Don't mess with the pancreas," and "A fool with a tool is still a fool." While sayings such as these harbor important truths, perhaps the most honest is the expression that states, "The only way to avoid complications is to avoid operating." Put more bluntly, complications are an inevitable part of our careers as surgeons. And though the effects may range from uncomfortable to life-altering for both patients and providers, facing complications is an integral part of our education and growth.

Throughout both literature and common lexicon, the concepts of complications and medical errors are often conflated. For the broader medical community, a complication or adverse event may be defined as *a known and unavoidable risk of medical care*, while a medical error describes an *avoidable commission or omission* which may have negative consequences. However, as surgeons, what we commonly refer to as complications—instances like anastomotic leaks, postoperative hemorrhage, and wound infections—encompass both the above definitions. Thus, we more commonly separate complications into disease related (unavoidable) and provider related (avoidable). Yet, as all who have attended an M&M conference can attest, these distinctions are rarely cut and dried, as most complications can be attributed to a combination of patient-, provider-, and system-based factors.

While it is crucial to review and discuss these contributing factors, what is arguably more important is the way in which we react to complications. When we make mistakes, or patients have bad outcomes, it is important to remember that our

A. Brackett (✉)
ChristianaCare Health System, Newark, DE, USA
e-mail: arielle.brackett@christianacare.org

responsibility is first and foremost to our patients. As an intern placing a subclavian line in the ICU, I dropped a lung. I shamefully gathered the supplies to place a left chest tube, expecting my supervising chief to take over. However, he dismissed my suggestion, telling me, "This is your patient, your complication, and you are going to take care of what needs to be done." I will never forget that lesson in patient ownership. However, our duty to our patients does not end with performing an indicated procedure or intervention, but also includes having an honest conversation to disclose the error that occurred and discuss a plan forward. As trainees, we do not often receive formal instruction on error disclosure, which can make this process more stressful. The simplest approach is to honestly explain to patients and their families what happened, how it happened, and the future implications for the patient's health while genuinely expressing remorse and offering a sincere apology. Like most skills we acquire during our training, these conversations are something that require practice and should be experiences we lean in to as learners.

Although often less obvious, complications can also deeply affect caregivers, especially surgical trainees, who may be the "second victims" in these circumstances. The guilt we feel for the harm we have caused our patients, as well as fears regarding loss of reputation and possible litigation, can increase symptoms of burnout, depression, and PTSD. As such, it is imperative that we develop coping strategies which will allow us to face and overcome complications. Sometimes, this may mean unpacking a challenging case with coresidents and/or attendings you trust to help put the event in perspective and identify opportunities for improvement moving forward. This may also mean talking openly with your patient and their families to help you find closure. It is important to allow yourself to process the emotions that come from a challenging patient outcome, be it through conversations with colleagues, friends, and family, or even professional help.

Ultimately, we must accept the truth that we, as humans and surgical trainees, are imperfect and prone to mistakes. We can and should do our best to prevent and mitigate them, but we cannot expect to avoid them completely. Instead, we must remember to lean into discomfort and learn every day.

Pearls
- We, as humans and surgical trainees, are imperfect and prone to mistakes.
- The most important part in disclosure of a medical error is your apology.
- We grow by leaning into discomfort and learning every day.

Chapter 35
Dealing with the Difficult Patient

Praveen Satarasinghe

You walk into a new patient's room amidst an entire list of patients, a full day in the operating room, and an endless list of tasks. The patient is complaining of a hernia that protrudes from his abdomen, but the patient continues to actively smoke tobacco and drink alcohol in addition to having a list of comorbidities including diabetes, hypertension, heart failure, chronic kidney disease, hyperlipidemia, and prior cardiac and abdominal surgeries—for all of which he has a laundry list of medications, which he does not take. As a busy resident, you efficiently allocate your time and decide to convince the patient to prepare for surgery; however, when you start to mention the medications and preoperative preparation required, you are greeted with indifference and negativity. He does not want to stop smoking, he does not want to take his medications, he has no way of getting to your office for surgery after being discharged, he has no place to go after surgery, he has low medical literacy, and he belligerently threatens you that he will take legal action if he does not get the surgery or if the surgery goes poorly. You investigate the charts, and the patient has had hospitalizations for similar issues in the past. Having sworn to the Hippocratic oath, your duty as a surgical resident is to respect the patient's desires and move forward with beneficence. This illustrative case is an example of a difficult patient from a multitude of lenses. In this chapter, an effective method for dealing with these numerous challenges of working with a difficult patient will be explained.

The first difficulty in treating the patient described in the vignette is *resistance*. When walking into a room, a patient notices every action that a physician makes. Body language when entering a room and working with a difficult patient are key to establishing a friendly patient-surgeon relationship [1] (Fig. 35.1). The most

P. Satarasinghe (✉)
Crozer Medical Center, Upland, PA, USA
e-mail: praveen.satarasinghe@crozer.org

© The Author(s), under exclusive license to Springer Nature
Switzerland AG 2023
A. Ratnasekera et al. (eds.), *General Surgery Residency Survival Guide*,
https://doi.org/10.1007/978-3-031-25617-2_35

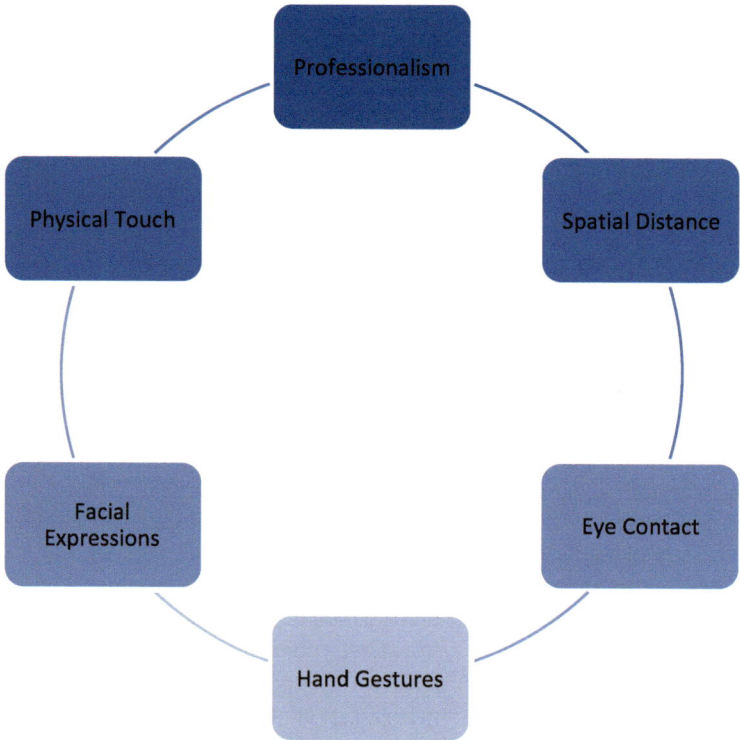

Fig. 35.1 Components of body language

effective patient-surgeon relationships start with forward-facing eye and body contact. Rather than speaking to the wall while standing, a better approach is to sit down and engage the patient's gaze with a calm, collected presence. A body can help convey a message that words cannot solely tell. With a difficult patient, it is easy to erupt and blame the patient or walk out of the room without thinking about how to best help the patient. It is important to recognize your own triggers as a resident and try to correct your body language to a manner that shows patience, engagement, and curiosity in the patient's needs.

Along with body language, residents must learn not to get defensive themselves and not to make assumptions about the origin of the patient's defensive attitude [2]. Keeping an objective perspective and focusing on the solution and treatment of the patient rather than the barriers of the personality will help you always respond with care and concern. Amidst being angry, most difficult patients will open up to reveal their story with positive body language. After providing time and attention, a sense of trust is created, and the difficult patient will let down his or her resistant curtain and reveal an inner fear that he or she now feels comfortable sharing with you.

Listening to a difficult patient rather than lecturing a difficult patient is the best approach. Frequent acknowledgements are an effective way of focusing attention and strengthening trust. Tell the patient that you understand his or her concern. Ask questions about how you can best respond to his or her concerns. Though the patient remains at the center, it is equally important to set boundaries with difficult patients. Walking out without assessing the situation properly is an immature and ineffective response. However, after deploying the strategies noted above, if a difficult patient continues to be irate, ending a consultation is appropriate. Sometimes, it is more effective to try again the next day or take a break and reattempt creating the patient-surgeon relationship when the patient is calm or when your thoughts as a surgeon are collected.

In my short time as a surgical resident, I have also learned the utility of informal and formal patient satisfaction surveys when working with difficult patients. Most of the time, difficult patients just want to be heard (Table 35.1). By providing a survey for written feedback, a difficult patient's concerns can be conveyed with the rest of the healthcare team [3]. Writing thoughts can sometimes be a better form of initial communication in a tense situation. Lastly, tackling resistance comes down to proactivity. Difficult patients who come back with the same issues every month are unlikely to suddenly change after a single interaction. Constant de-escalation techniques, frequent feedback, and incorporation of the above methods in a proactive yet reasonable manner will transform patient resistance into openness.

The second difficulty in treating the difficult patient in the initial situation is *somatization.* Many difficult patients will present with multiple medical issues and noncompliance with treatment plans and will try to threaten the care plan with vague complaints and symptoms that do not align with clinical presentation [4]. Often, the difficulty of somatization can be resolved with a thorough explanation of the diagnosis and treatment plan in an empathetic fashion. The vague complaints and symptoms may not be the result of ill-minded goals, but rather unfamiliarity with the disease process. By explaining that certain symptoms are unrelated and certain symptoms are related, the difficult patient will have an objective set of information. Whether the difficult patient uses the information positively may be up in the air. However, taking the time to provide information may gain the trust of the difficult patient, rather than an argument with an abrupt ending. In the hospital setting, I have also encountered difficult patients bouncing from one hospital to another. Rather than trying to send a difficult patient to another provider, the most effective method of handling somatization is trying to treat the patient under one hospital team or physician. Continuity of care is created, the difficult patient feels more connected to the surgical team, and problems can be solved rather than restarting with

Table 35.1 Factors that were recognized by patients as important in surgical care	
	1. Personalized care plan
	2. Multiple options for treatment—operative/non-operative
	3. Next steps/coordination of care with other specialists
	4. Simplified communication with surgery steps
	5. Good listening skills/taking time
	6. Well informed/Educated surgeon

the complete history and physical at a new location. This would mitigate the frustration of acclimating to an unfamiliar health system, new medical team, and travel to an unfamiliar health system. Lastly, somatization can be countered by scheduling follow-up appointments that are brief. Difficult patients often list many reasons for their problems. However, by establishing brief, frequent, efficient visits, one complaint at a time can be handled—preventing accumulated frustration on both the surgeon and patient sides.

The third difficulty in treating the difficult patient in the initial situation is *manipulation*. As explained before, the key to tackling manipulation is to have the confidence to say "no" in a respective manner that will not break the patient-surgeon bond. Saying "no" can become more comfortable by establishing a partnership with the patient and the surgical resident striving for the same goal [5, 6]. Being aware of one's own emotions and goals in the patient interaction will make this task easier. With manipulation, a difficult patient can also divide staff members. When multiple care team members are involved, it is important to have everyone on the same page and not to have one party apologize and one party accept every need of the patient. Difficult patients manipulate because of the need for attention, desire to feel important, possible personality disorders, and limited social interactions with others. The need for these social desires can be provided by presenting yourself as a surgical resident professionally, giving the patient choices, and asking questions that will focus the spotlight on the patient.

The fourth and last difficulty in treating the difficult patient comes with *medical complexity*. Of the four described challenges of working with a difficult patient, this may be less difficult to tackle. Just as in communicating complex medical problems with a patient, treating a complex medical problem requires assessing the information and establishing a step-by-step plan rather than solving every problem all at once.

As described above, the difficult patient comes with a variety of issues that need to be tackled. Though the word "difficult" is attached to the patient, both patient factors and physician factors contribute to tackling (1) resistance, (2) somatization, (3) manipulation, and (4) medical complexity—a quartet of traits displayed by the difficult patient. Surgical residents need to focus on self-management in addition to acknowledging the patient. Difficult patients require time and attention. The healthcare system may not provide the best environment for allowing a physician to work with difficult patients with a lack of resources and time. The US healthcare system is filled with high costs of care, lack of insurance coverage, lack of transparency, poor empowerment of physicians, and dysfunctional scheduling goals driven by quantity over quality. Despite the improperly built healthcare network, our goal as physicians and surgeons should always be to use communication techniques that strengthen the patient-practitioner relationship and allow greater patient involvement in their care.

Pearls
- A multimodal approach must be utilized to deal with a difficult patient.
- Body language is an important aspect during patient discussions.
- Focus on the problem at hand rather than the personality barriers.
- Take time to explain the diagnosis, treatment plan, and medications.

References

1. Berman AC, Chutka DS. Assessing effective physician-patient communication skills: "are you listening to me, doc?". Korean J Med Educ. 2016;28(2):243–9. https://doi.org/10.3946/kjme.2016.21.
2. Glass RM. The patient-physician relationship. JAMA focuses on the center of medicine. JAMA. 1996;275(2):147–8.
3. Meredith P. Patient satisfaction with communication in general surgery: problems of measurement and improvement. Soc Sci Med. 1993;37(5):591–602. https://doi.org/10.1016/0277-9536(93)90098-o.
4. Kleinsinger F. Working with the noncompliant patient. Perm J. 2010;14(1):54–60. https://doi.org/10.7812/TPP/09-064.
5. Reach G. Patient education, nudge, and manipulation: defining the ethical conditions of the person-centered model of care. Patient Prefer Adherence. 2016;10:459–68. Published 2016 Apr 4. https://doi.org/10.2147/PPA.S99627.
6. Carlsen B, Norheim OF. "Saying no is no easy matter" a qualitative study of competing concerns in rationing decisions in general practice. BMC Health Serv Res. 2005;5:70. Published 2005 Nov 9. https://doi.org/10.1186/1472-6963-5-70.

Chapter 36
The Difficult Attending

Sirivan Seng

A "difficult" attending can be deemed such for a variety of reasons. This overly subjective term is broad, and depending on the reason, the approach to a solution will differ greatly. All surgical residents at one time or another will encounter what one would consider a "difficult" attending. This can be minor as having high expectations, being extremely picky in the operating room, and micromanaging patient care, to egregious acts such as intimidation, occupational sabotage, verbal abuse, physical abuse, or refusing to allow specific residents operate with them. A national survey administered after an annual surgical in-training exam in 2018 found that residents reported attendings as the source of 52.4% of verbal or emotional abuse, 19.8% of gender discrimination, 17.4% of racial discrimination, 21.7% of physical abuse, 27.2% of sexual harassment, and 36.8% of pregnancy or childcare discrimination [1].

Managing Interactions with the Difficult Attending

When faced with an attending who is difficult because of perceived high expectations, being particular in the operating room or with patient care, it is vital to keep a few things in mind. Take this criticism with a smile. It is important to stay focused and keep an open mind to be able to empathize with where your attending is coming from. Try to discern their motivations so that you can anticipate their expectations and identify any triggers that may cause any grief. It is additionally vital that you self-reflect and realize if you have made a mistake. Overall, it is important to stay professional and not let your interaction with your attending affect your work,

S. Seng (✉)
Crozer Chester Medical Center, Upland, PA, USA
e-mail: sirivan.seng@crozer.org

A. Ratnasekera et al. (eds.), *General Surgery Residency Survival Guide*,
https://doi.org/10.1007/978-3-031-25617-2_36

thereby negatively affecting patient care. Talk to your colleagues and senior residents. They have had the time to learn how to mitigate these situations and have survived. Know that conflict within the workplace over the course of 5 years is almost inevitable.

Should you face the "difficult" attending who commits acts of intimidation, occupational sabotage, and verbal or physical abuse, let your senior residents, mentor, or program director know [2]. Remember that you have many people advocating for you, your educational success, and emotional well-being. Your program director is there to help you and acts as a mediator between residents, attendings, and the rest of the hospital. The culture of surgical training is changing, and there is a growing intolerance for abusive and intimidating behaviors.

As someone who went through multiple years of preliminary surgical training, I have felt particularly vulnerable to the "difficult" attending. Just coming out of medical school, it was almost impossible for me to discern from the overly critical attending to one who was committing acts of intimidation and occupational sabotage. During my third month of my preliminary surgical year, I had been placed in the surgical intensive care unit as the only resident. I was charged that day to wean sedation from an intubated patient and prepare to extubate. As with many young trauma patients, this patient was extremely agitated and combative and I did not know how to proceed. I called my attending for assistance who then proceeded to berate me for even considering calling him for such a low-priority issue and hung up the phone. He then called me back a few moments later to again berate and tell me that this was why interns should not be in the intensive care unit. The next day, during our surgical morbidity and mortality conference, he publicly berated me for the same issue. This continued in private and public settings for much of my preliminary surgical year where sometimes I was cornered into private spaces to be verbally abused. Being yelled at and humiliated in such a manner caused me to feel helpless and shy away from asking for help during my rotations out of fear of repercussions. This could have caused harm to my patients and impacted my surgical education. Unfortunately, as a preliminary surgical resident, I often felt like I needed to avoid making waves, prove myself, and appear more confident and able than I was, so I never turned to my program director, other attendings, friends, or family for help with this matter. Looking back after all these years, I wish I had the courage to handle that situation differently and reached out to people that I felt comfortable with for help and guidance [3]. If I did, I could have likely had a different outcome from that training year or at least remember it much more fondly than that of which I am writing to you now.

> The other people with whom you interact are mirrors that help you see things within yourself. With some people, that mirror can be difficult to view, yet when you have the courage to do so, the rewards can be many and great.—Ralph Marston

Pearls
- Even the most difficult of attendings has something to teach you.
- Seek advice from those who have come before you.
- Reach out to your program director; they are the intermediary between residents and attendings.

References

1. Hu YY, Ellis RJ, Hewitt DB, Yang AD, Cheung EO, Moskowitz JT, Potts JR 3rd, Buyske J, Hoyt DB, Nasca TJ, Bilimoria KY. Discrimination, abuse, harassment, and burnout in surgical residency training. N Engl J Med. 2019;381(18):1741–52. https://doi.org/10.1056/NEJMsa1903759. Epub 2019 Oct 28
2. Hall A. Encounters with difficult bosses: how do you cope? Biomed Instrum Technol. 2007;41(1):45–7. https://doi.org/10.2345/0899-8205(2007)41[45:ewdbhd]2.0.co;2.
3. Overton AR, Lowry AC. Conflict management: difficult conversations with difficult people. Clin Colon Rectal Surg. 2013;26(4):259–64. https://doi.org/10.1055/s-0033-1356728.

Chapter 37
How to Be Empathetic

James Jarvis

Introduction

Empathy can be defined as "the action of understanding, being aware of, being sensitive to, and vicariously experiencing the feelings, thoughts, and experience of another [...]" [1]. Despite a universal sense of empathy being one of the defining characteristics of a physician and surgeon, residency training programs often do not offer structured training or didactics in the instruction of empathy. In fact, evidence points towards a decline in empathy throughout the process of medical training, which begins during the clinical years of medical school and continues through postgraduate training [2]. This chapter addresses the importance of empathy as an essential attribute for surgeons and highlights strategies to maintain empathy during the hardships of training.

When you think of what defines a capable, well-respected surgeon, which qualities come to mind? Good technical skill, strong focus, and unwavering commitment are certainly necessary inherent traits in a surgical trainee in order to succeed through difficult surgical training. However, another indispensable characteristic of physicians, and especially surgeons, is empathy. Empathy, as defined above, allows surgeons to relate with their patients, build stronger relationships, derive better job satisfaction, and may even improve patient outcomes [3]. Emotional intelligence, another crucially important attribute of surgeons, relates to the ability to assess and regulate emotions during patient encounters—a skill that can be equally important to surgeons as steady handedness. One investigation that surveyed surgeons and their patients undergoing surgery found that surgeons with a higher emotional intelligence were more likely to have improved patient satisfaction scores and better patient self-reported outcomes after surgery [4].

J. Jarvis (✉)
ChristianaCare Health System, Newark, DE, USA
e-mail: james.m.jarvis@christianacare.org

© The Author(s), under exclusive license to Springer Nature Switzerland AG 2023
A. Ratnasekera et al. (eds.), *General Surgery Residency Survival Guide*,
https://doi.org/10.1007/978-3-031-25617-2_37

Compared to other medical specialties, surgery has additional challenging demands, which place the development and practice of empathy at a disadvantage—the procedural aspect, exposure to pain and trauma, and steep learning curve. This, coupled with the need for decisive action and quick thinking, makes empathy a daunting skill to utilize in surgical training. One could also argue that in a training environment such as the one that exists today, with poor work-life balance, mistreatment, and rampant burnout, it is increasingly difficult to demonstrate empathy due to multiple stressors on trainees.

What can we, as surgical trainees, do to improve our own empathy in our interactions with patients? Many residency programs have attempted to incorporate communication-based instruction, including breaking bad news, disclosing complications, etc. in an attempt to "teach empathy" [5]. If your training program has this incorporated into the curriculum, utilize these sessions to learn these important "nontechnical" skills. Practice with your peers with role-playing scenarios, including delivering bad news and dealing with the "difficult patient."

Another method to learn how empathy can be used in the busy daily work of a surgeon is to identify a role model that you identify with personally and learn to model the positive aspects of their empathic interactions with patients. Of course, one potential downside to this method is that selected mentors may not demonstrate best practices, so you must be mindful of your selection.

In addition, before you are able to exhibit empathic communication towards your patients, you must also allow time for self-reflection and mindfulness, both of which are helpful in addressing burnout. Daily meditation, introspection, and self-care (exercise, time with family, de-stressing activities) are essential to your longevity as a physician and surgeon. You must provide adequate care for yourself before you can appropriately care for others.

Pearls
- Empathy is the ability to understand and relate to others without necessarily having lived through their experiences.
- Emotional intelligence, the ability to perceive and regulate emotion, is an extremely valuable skill that must be honed to maximize patient encounters, especially difficult ones.
- Take advantage of expanding surgical residency curricula in "nontechnical skills," such as empathy, and practice with your peers.
- Identify surgical role models who demonstrate good empathic communication with their patients.
- You must show empathy to yourself during the hardships of surgical training before you can demonstrate it to your patients.

References

1. Merriam-Webster (n.d.) Empathy. In Merriam-Webster.com dictionary. Retrieved 18 June 2022 from https://www.merriam-webster.com/dictionary/empathy
2. Han J, Pappas T. A review of empathy, its importance, and its teaching in surgical training. J Surg Educ. 2017;75:88.
3. Hojat M, Louis D, Markham F, Wender R, Rabinowitz C, Gonnella J. Physicians' empathy and clinical outcomes for diabetic patients. Acad Med. 2011;86:359.
4. Weng H, Steed J, Yu S, Liu Y, Hsu C, Yu T, Chen W. The effect of surgeon empathy and emotional intelligence on patient satisfaction. Adv in Health Sci Educ, vol. 16; 2011. p. 591.
5. Kapadia M, Lee E, Healy H, Dort J, Rosenbaum M, Newcomb A. Training surgical residents to communicated with their patients: a scoping review of the literature. J Surg Educ. 2020;78:440.

Chapter 38
"Just Another Day in Paradise": The Emotional Trash Compactor of Residency

Bradford Bormann

In my experience, workplaces and professions where employees maintain a common disposition are like giant trash compactors. You, a shiny, unique vehicle, are placed within the confines of the compactor with the iron walls slowly approaching you, steel scraping along massive hydraulic pistons. The walls make contact with you, applying ever-mounting pressure. Your joints and facets hold fast at first, before buckling under the stress. Soon your structure is collapsing inwards, ever closer to the form of the other vehicles that have been there longer than you. Eventually, you are another cube, of equal volume and appearance to all the others. Perhaps you are even looking back at the next model getting placed eagerly onto the compactor, waiting for the validation of it getting crushed down to size as well. Slowly, the common culture of the hospital has eroded you towards mild bitterness, skepticism, and chronic exhaustion, an emotional cube all too similar to the ones on either side.

An example from my intern year: I was covering the trauma pager, and a patient with a well-documented history of struggling with intravenous drug addiction and AMA discharge was threatening to leave the hospital. Despite my most empathic efforts, I could not compel her to stay with us a little longer to control pain from her tibia-fibula fracture. She looked me in the eyes, uttered an unsavory phrase, packed her bags, and pushed past me, hobbling on an air cast. Two hours later, she was back in the ED, tearful and apologetic, one more consult to churn through.

The hospital is a powerful trash compactor applying unrelenting pressure. Endless geriatric patients on blood thinners who fall from standing. The patient presenting with their 11th SBO. Residents, nurses, and support staff all chafing against burnout. To some extent, we all get crushed down into cubes. Here is my advice on this:

B. Bormann (✉)
ChristianaCare Health System, Newark, DE, USA
e-mail: bradford.bormann@christianacare.org

Give into the compactor a little bit. Becoming a cube is participating in the culture of your program and profession and will help you empathize with your colleagues. If we ever want to change to a compactor—or perhaps the shapes it forms us into—knowing the pressures it applies is a critical first step.

Bring more cubes in at once! As one vehicle, it is nigh on impossible to resist the clamp of the walls. However, bringing more cubes onto the floor can help keep the walls at bay. That is: empathize with your colleagues. No one should go through this alone. Working to support and sustain one another, to become aware of insidious frustrations, countertransference, and patient prejudice, is critical.

Do not stop the walls—stop the engine. Certainly easier said than done. Fighting the walls is impossible. No one can deliver that much resistance for so long. But you CAN pull the plug. Or remove gas from the tank. Or whatever you need to do to shut down a trash compactor. What is the root of the issue applying pressure? What is/are the seminal causes for your everyday issues? Reading and understanding about the sources of your frustration is a great way to develop empathy—as well as a vision for how these frustrations can be changed.

Pearls
- Understanding the culture of your residency program and institution may help you develop ideas for change.
- Utilizing your colleagues for support during the long journey is imperative.

Part V
Basic Survival Skills

Chapter 39
The Benefits of Sleep

Madelyn Hernandez

Introduction

I once heard an Irish proverb: "A good laugh and a long sleep are the best cures in the doctor's book." As I heard this quote, and reflected on its meaning, I thought to myself; as healthcare professionals, we may preach this, but it is definitely not what we practice. Sleep is a universal process, and it connects us all as beings. Why do we do it? Why do we need it for survival? These are just a few questions that many scientists have pondered over the years. With research, we have come to learn a few things about this topic, but there is still much that is unclear about sleep, the processes that occur in our brains and bodies during this state of being, and how it affects our day-to-day life.

The Science of Sleep

In order to understand something better, we need to learn the science, research, and history of that topic. So … what is sleep and how is it different from the awake state? Sleep is not a passive state of being. It is a metabolically active state that is essential for health and well-being. Scientists have described specific neurochemical pathways in our brains that are involved in the processes that maintain wakefulness named the "ascending arousal system." This system consists of many different regions in the brain and different neurochemicals, which play specific roles in keeping us awake. A few of these include norepinephrine from the locus coeruleus,

M. Hernandez (✉)
Christiana Care Health System, Newark, DE, USA
e-mail: madelyn.b.hernandez@christianacare.org

A. Ratnasekera et al. (eds.), *General Surgery Residency Survival Guide*,
https://doi.org/10.1007/978-3-031-25617-2_39

serotonin from the midline raphe nuclei, histamine from the tuberomammillary nucleus, and many others. Normal awake behavior requires all of these arousing systems to function properly. On the contrary, sleep then requires suppression of the activity in this ascending arousal system, which is accomplished by inhibitory neurons of the ventrolateral preoptic area. Essentially, sleep and wake states are controlled by the proper functioning and appropriate inhibiting of the ascending arousal system [1].

As the sleep state begins, there are different processes that occur. Combined, these processes make up a sleep period. There are two fundamentally distinct types of sleep: rapid eye movement (REM) sleep, which is associated with active dreaming, and non-rapid eye movement (NREM) sleep, which is associated with reduced skeletal muscle tone. Alternations between NREM and REM sleep are controlled by neurons in the brain stem. This results in the cycling between NREM and REM during the sleep period. There are three stages of NREM sleep: N1 is the lightest stage of NREM sleep; N2 sleep is the in-between stage; and N3 is the deepest stage of NREM sleep. As mentioned previously, the sleep process is cyclical. After the onset of sleep, we quickly flow through the N1 and N2 stages and enter the deep-sleep stage N3 within the first hour. This is followed by cyclical alternations between NREM and REM every 60–90 min. The majority of our deep NREM sleep occurs during the first half of the sleep period, and the majority of REM sleep occurs during the second half of the sleep period. Individuals will undergo about 4–6 cyclical alterations during a sleep period, which results in a full night's sleep cycle [1]. REM sleep is the major source of dreams. NREM sleep is associated with variable processes such as growth hormone secretion and brain metabolite clearance. The full function of sleep has not been fully elucidated, although it is considered to be important for body restitution, memory consolidation, energy conservation, thermoregulation, and tissue recovery [2].

In this day and age, the topic of sleep is a peculiar one. Some people anecdotally claim only needing 3–5 hours of sleep a night, while others insist on requiring at least 8 hours or more of sleep per night for optimal performance. How much sleep is too little or too much? Sleep deficiency is when you sleep for less than what your body needs or if the sleep quality is suboptimal [3]. Sleep deprivation is when we are unable to meet the biological requirement of sleep. This can be acute, chronic, partial, or total. Total sleep deprivation is eliminating sleep for one night in order to prolong wakefulness. There is no doubt that many of us have partaken in this at least a few times during our education and training. I can remember a few all-nighters I pulled to cram for exams and finals. Partial sleep deprivation is reducing the amount of sleep one has in a night. When partial sleep deprivation occurs over extended periods of time, this is known as chronic sleep deprivation [4].

There are many contributing factors to sleep deficiency including occupational commitments societal demands, psychiatric or physical disorders, environmental factors, and others. Whether we are aware of it or not, society places an emphasis on certain values, one of which is success. A universal life goal is to be successful. While the average American gets 6 hours and 51 minutes of sleep a night, some people think that by sleeping less, there is extra time for work. Time is an essential commodity and how it is used determines if and how you will be successful. Although less sleep equates to more time spared for other activities, this does not necessarily equate to a more productive use of that spare time. It is a common misconception that busy productive people need less sleep. This fallacy is perpetuated by individuals in the workforce who set poor examples for their employees to follow. Individuals that sleep for more than 6 hours or partake in naps during the day are at times considered "lazy." As working professionals, it has been ingrained in us that sleep can be sacrificed and is not necessary for our overall well-being. In fact, people often boast about the little hours of sleep they need, implying that less sleep equates to higher productivity. How little sleep we need has become a symbol of our prowess, prioritizing work over health and wellness.

One can argue that sleeping less does allow for more "free time" during a 24-hour day. While this is true from a numbers standpoint, that does not mean that extra time is being put to good use. In a study performed by Ericsson et al. (1993) observing the role of deliberate practice on mastering musical performance versus the role of innate talent, they found that deliberate and intense practice was the most common factor among the musical geniuses. They also found that in addition to practice, sleep was another activity shown to be essential and prioritized in these maestros. The average amount of sleep these maestros participated in was 8 hours and 36 minutes per night. This is about 100 more minutes per night than the average individual [5]. Another study by Coleman (1986) showed that Olympic athletes sleep close to 8 hours a night and take an additional half-hour nap each day [6]. From these studies, one can deduce that these champions in their respective fields do not sacrifice sleep but in fact prioritize sleep, and as a result reap the benefits of having a good night's rest.

If top performers in different fields prioritize sleep, then why do medical health professionals not do the same? For anyone going through the schooling and training to become a nurse, physician assistant, or doctor, you know the toll it can take physically, mentally, psychologically, and emotionally for many years. Specifically, the journey to become a physician includes 4 years of undergraduate school, 4 years of medical school, then 2–7 years of residency depending on the specialty of choice, possibly followed by 1+ years of fellowship training. That equates to 10+ years of strenuous mental focus, late-night study sessions, poor sleep hygiene, and subpar nutrition. People in healthcare tend to stretch their capacity and compromise their nightly sleep, thus becoming sleep deprived. The cumulative effects of work-related sleep deprivation can affect cognitive performance immensely. Studies have shown that decreased sleep affects higher order cognitive tasks [7]. As sleep is diminished, tasks requiring judgment are impaired and therefore increasingly risky behaviors emerge. Small amounts of sleep loss (e.g., 1 hour per night over several nights) have subtle cognitive effects, while more severe sleep deprivation for a week or more can result in profound cognitive deficits similar to those seen in stroke patients [8].

Medical professionals, and specifically resident physicians who are involved in long-term night-shift schedules during their postgraduate training, are prone to acute and chronic sleep deprivation and disruption, putting them at risk for medical errors. In a study by Choshen-Hillel et al. (2021), medical students and residents were evaluated twice—once at baseline and once after a 26-hour shift. They underwent computerized tests of attention and behavior, completed a risk-taking questionnaire, and answered a sleep quality index. Residents reported chronic sleep deprivation and showed impaired global executive function, increased impulsivity, and slower processing times [9]. Another study compared post-call performance during a heavy call rotation (every fourth or fifth night) to performance with blood alcohol concentration of 0.04–0.05 g% and found them to be comparable in sustained attention, vigilance, and simulated tasks. Sleep loss and alcohol use can essentially affect tasks in a similar way [10]. A study published in the *Lancet* examined the effect of sleep deprivation on surgical manual dexterity. Surgical skills were tested with a laparoscopic surgery simulator in six residents under three conditions: undisturbed night of sleep, a night on call with three disturbances, and a night with no sleep. The study reports that surgeons who had not slept made 20% more errors and took 14% longer to complete the tasks than those who had a full night's sleep [11]. This highlights the impairment of neurobehavioral performance due to extended work hours, increased risk for medical errors, and serious implications for patient safety.

Sleep is one aspect of our well-being that affects all elements in our lives. If we get adequate sleep, our decision-making, creativity, judgment, and performance all improve. Lack of sleep does the complete opposite. Not only does sleep deprivation affect cognition, but it also affects your weight and mood, increases your risk of diabetes and cardiovascular disease, and even negatively affects your skin. According to a 2004 study, people who sleep less than 6 hours a day are more than 30% more likely to become obese [12]. Another study shows that sufficient sleep helps your body process glucose. People who persistently sleep less than 5 hours a night have bodies that do not perform this function effectively, placing these individuals at risk for prediabetes or type II diabetes [13].

Lack of sleep can lead to burnout and influence your mood [14]. People are more likely to experience anxiety and/or depression with lack of sleep and are up to five times more likely to develop depression [15]. The results of a survey given to interns before their internship began and again during their internship found that depression rates were highest among interns with sleep disturbances and sleep deprivation. The study also found that medical error rates were higher when the interns slept less than 6 hours per night and worked more than 70 hours per week [16]. Not only is the importance on the total sleep time, but also factors such as later bedtime, earlier wake time, and variable sleep have been associated with increased depression among medical trainees [17].

Not only has sleep loss been linked to anxiety, depression, and even diabetes, but sleep deficiency also interferes with so many aspects of day-to-day life and health. Researchers at Duke University Medical Center found that poor sleep is associated with greater psychological distress and higher levels of biomarkers associated with elevated risk of heart disease, associations which were significantly stronger in women than in men [18]. Lastly, without an adequate amount of sleep, your body releases more of the stress hormone cortisol. In excess amounts, cortisol breaks down skin collagen, the protein that keeps skin smooth and elastic, resulting in higher risk of poor skin texture and wrinkles [19].

Now that we have reviewed the importance of sleep, and the consequences that manifest with sleep deficiency, how can we change our current sleep habits to optimize our lives and reap the benefits of sleep? First you need to figure out what your optimal sleep time is. This can be accomplished by going to sleep at the same time every night for a few days and then allowing yourself to wake up in the morning naturally without any alarm clocks. After repeating this for ~5–7 days, you can determine your minimum sleep time, aka how much sleep you need in a given night to feel rested in the morning. Certain professions make this homework a bit more challenging. One suggestion is to do this during a vacation week. After you have determined the minimum amount of sleep you need in a night, you can adjust your bedtime to maximize your sleep schedule. For example, let us say that you notice your body wakes up naturally after 7 and half hours of sleep. This becomes your sleep threshold. If you need to wake up at 6 am to be at work by 7 am, your bedtime should be set for 10:30 pm in order to obtain the full 7.5 hours of sleep you need.

Now let us talk about caffeine. Caffeine is one of the most widely consumed stimulants in the world, with about 90% of Americans consuming a caffeine beverage at least once daily. We all know about the enhancing performance of caffeine, but there are negative effects with caffeine as well. Caffeine has a half-life of 6 hours. This means that if someone consumes a cup of coffee at noon, by 6 pm there is still half the dose of caffeine in that person's system, and by midnight there is still 25% of that caffeine dose flowing through their bloodstream. The presence of caffeine in your system will interfere with your sleep/wake cycle and result in sleep disturbances. This does not mean that you are no longer allowed to take your daily dose of caffeine. In order to optimize your sleep schedule, consider having your coffee early in the morning and limit your intake later in the day by replacing a caffeinated beverage with a decaffeinated option [20].

Combating fatigue is an issue that is common across many professions that work days and nights. Implementing strategies to mitigate fatigue and promote alertness can be beneficial for performance, productivity, and safety. One strategy that has been shown to be effective in improving performance and alertness is taking naps. Not only are naps beneficial for toddlers in daycare, but adults can benefit from naps, too. A 1995 study from the US National Aeronautics and Space Administration (NASA) found that a 26-minute nap improves performance by 34% and alertness by 54%. Although the benefits of naps have been shown in several studies, there is a risk of disrupting nighttime sleep cycles with longer naps of more than 30 minutes. Biohackers have managed to control their nap time and use them during the most optimal time, in the early afternoon, in order to optimize their performance and maintain alertness for longer periods in the day. By setting aside some time and implementing 26-minutes naps during the workday, colleagues can combat fatigue and ultimately improve task performance [21].

Being in the medical field and working as a healthcare provider, we desire to have all the answers to our patients' problems and be able to offer a helpful solution. At times, the "help" we give is only putting a Band-Aid over the wound, providing temporary relief but not a long-lasting solution. For example, some people would think that the remedy for abnormal sleep would be to take a sleep aid or a sleeping pill. Sometimes, the norm in Western medicine is to prescribe a medication as a temporary fix to any ailment. Although some conditions require the use of medications as the gold standard of treatment, not all disorders or deficiencies require medications. In fact, patients with sleep deficiencies or disorders may not benefit from medications and the use of medications can potentially result in more harmful effects. Medications can also become addictive at times and are no longer helpful. Promoting good sleep hygiene is more beneficial and longer lasting than any temporary elixir or pill.

So what is good sleep hygiene? It is a collection of behaviors, lifestyle, and environmental conditions that aim to ensure good-quality sleep. Common sleep hygiene behaviors include optimizing the bedroom environment by ensuring a cool, dark, and quiet setting, minimizing light or devices such as laptops or cell phones before bedtime, and avoiding alcohol, caffeine, or strenuous exercise before bed. In a 2022 study by Rampling et al., researchers found that having engagement in sleep hygiene practices was associated with better sleep quality [22].

Over the last few years, society has shed a spotlight on the importance of wellness and the harmful effects of burnout found in the healthcare industry. Sleep deprivation and burnout are widespread in healthcare workers, affecting nurses, medical students, physician assistants, physicians in training, and practicing physicians. Nearly 50% of physicians report symptoms of clinical burnout [19]. It has been a goal to identify effective solutions and interventions to promote resiliency among healthcare trainees. One study examined the impact of app-delivered mindfulness meditation on self-reported mental health symptoms among physician assistant students. Surprisingly, they found that the mindfulness group reported improvements in sleep impairment [23]. Essentially, mindfulness was found as an effective tool to improve sleep dysfunction in medical health trainees. While many more studies will need to be conducted in order to elucidate the effects of mindfulness on other aspects of life, using mindfulness on a regular basis and incorporating meditation into practice can help healthcare providers with their mental health and improve their overall sleep hygiene [13].

Although many, if not all, of these strategies have been shown to improve sleep quality, the importance of improving sleep is still not a standard or a priority among healthcare professionals. The Accreditation Council for Graduate Medical Education now limits resident work hours to 80 hours per week (double what the average employed American works on a weekly basis) [24]. Curtailing resident work hours has been seen as a positive and a negative in the healthcare field. On the one hand, placing work hour limits results in more time for rest and a better work-life balance. On the other hand, working less hours results in decreased continuity of patient care and decreased time to learn the profession. Medical professionals that trained prior to the ACGME work-hour limitations viewed the arduous training schedule as a rite of passage and prepare trainees for the workplace. Lastly, the more hours trainees and residents work, the more money it saves the teaching hospitals [11]. Changing the culture of an institution that has been in place for many years is not an overnight occurrence. As more awareness is placed on the importance of mitigating fatigue in the workplace, increased buy-in will result in cultural change over time.

Identifying sleep abnormalities by institutions can lead to the early identification of individuals in the healthcare field at risk for sleep deprivation and its dangerous consequences. Implementing programs that educate employees and promote healthy sleep practices can lead to minimization and hopefully prevention of fatigue and clinical burnout. Optimal schedules can be developed using the scientific data presented in this manuscript, including minimizing night/24-hour shifts, determining your sleep threshold and meeting that requirement nightly, maximizing sleep quality by optimizing sleep time and sleep hygiene, and lastly normalizing the importance of rest and sleep in the work environment leading to a culture that encourages and celebrates health and well-being.

One of the first things they teach us as we enter the medical field, and an important step we take to become a medical health professional, is taking the Hippocratic Oath. "First, Do no harm." This is the foundational pillar that medicine is built on. This phrase describes that as a medical professional, our goal is to serve our patients and to offer solutions to their problems without jeopardizing their health or causing more harm than good. I believe that this phrase should also be used as a motto for how we treat ourselves. As healthcare professionals, we oftentimes sacrifice our health and well-being for the benefit of others. As clinicians, we should take priority in our own health and well-being and strive to perform our best, to learn as much as we can, and to use that knowledge in the care of our patients.

Pearls
- It is important to understand the underlying physiology of sleep.
- Identify sleep abnormalities that may be affecting you.
- Adopt some strategies to improve your sleep habits.

References

1. Carley DW, Farabi SS. Physiology of sleep. Diabetes Spectr. 2016;29(1):5–9. https://doi.org/10.2337/diaspect.29.1.5.
2. Kashiwagi M, Hayashi Y. The function of REM sleep: implications from transgenic mouse models. Brain Nerve. 2016;68(10):1205–11. Japanese. https://doi.org/10.11477/mf.1416200575.
3. Gohari A, Baumann B, Jen R, Ayas N. Sleep deficiency: epidemiology and effects. Clin Chest Med. 2022;43(2):189–98. https://doi.org/10.1016/j.ccm.2022.02.001.
4. Buysse DJ. Sleep health: can we define it? Does it matter? Sleep. 2014;37(1):9–17. Published 2014 Jan 1. https://doi.org/10.5665/sleep.3298.
5. Ericsson KA, Krampe RT, Tesch-Römer C. The role of deliberate practice in the acquisition of expert performance. Psychol Rev. 1993;100(3):363–406. https://doi.org/10.1037/0033-295X.100.3.363.
6. Coleman RM. Wide awake at 3:00 A.M.: By choice or by chance. New York: W H Freeman/ Times Books/ Henry Holt & Co.; 1986.
7. Maquet P. The role of sleep in learning and memory. Science. 2001;294:1048–52.

8. Thorne D, Thomas M, Russo M, et al. Performance on a driving-simulator divided attention task during one week of restricted nightly sleep. Sleep. 1999;22(Suppl 1):301.
9. Choshen-Hillel S, Ishqer A, Mahameed F, Reiter J, Gozal D, Gileles-Hillel A, Berger I. Acute and chronic sleep deprivation in residents: cognition and stress biomarkers. Med Educ. 2021;55(2):174–84. https://doi.org/10.1111/medu.14296.
10. Arnedt JT, Owens J, Crouch M, Stahl J, Carskadon MA. Neurobehavioral performance of residents after heavy night call vs after alcohol ingestion. JAMA. 2005;294(9):1025–33. https://doi.org/10.1001/jama.294.9.1025.
11. Howard SK. Sleep deprivation and physician performance: why should I care? Proc (Bayl Univ Med Cent). 2005;18(2):108–13. https://doi.org/10.1080/08998280.2005.11928045.
12. Hasler G, Buysse DJ, Klaghofer R, Gamma A, Ajdacic V, Eich D, Rössler W, Angst J. The association between short sleep duration and obesity in young adults: a 13-year prospective study. Sleep. 2004;27(4):661–6. https://doi.org/10.1093/sleep/27.4.661.
13. Antza C, Kostopoulos G, Mostafa S, Nirantharakumar K, Tahrani A. The links between sleep duration, obesity and type 2 diabetes mellitus. J Endocrinol. 2021;252(2):125–41. https://doi.org/10.1530/JOE-21-0155.
14. Stewart NH, Arora VM. The impact of sleep and circadian disorders on physician burnout. Chest. 2019;156(5):1022–30. https://doi.org/10.1016/j.chest.2019.07.008.
15. Alhola P, Polo-Kantola P. Sleep deprivation: impact on cognitive performance. Neuropsychiatr Dis Treat. 2007;3(5):553–67.
16. Kalmbach DA, Arnedt JT, Song PX, Guille C, Sen S. Sleep disturbance and short sleep as risk factors for depression and perceived medical errors in first-year residents. Sleep. 2017;40(3):zsw073. https://doi.org/10.1093/sleep/zsw073.
17. Mansukhani MP, Kolla BP, Surani S, Varon J, Ramar K. Sleep deprivation in resident physicians, work hour limitations, and related outcomes: a systematic review of the literature. Postgrad Med. 2012;124(4):241–9. https://doi.org/10.3810/pgm.2012.07.2583.
18. Suarez EC. Self-reported symptoms of sleep disturbance and inflammation, coagulation, insulin resistance and psychosocial distress: evidence for gender disparity. Brain Behav Immun. 2008;22(6):960–8. https://doi.org/10.1016/j.bbi.2008.01.011.
19. Kahan V, Andersen ML, Tomimori J, Tufik S. Can poor sleep affect skin integrity? Med Hypotheses. 2010;75(6):535–7. https://doi.org/10.1016/j.mehy.2010.07.018.
20. O'Callaghan F, Muurlink O, Reid N. Effects of caffeine on sleep quality and daytime functioning. Risk Manag Healthc Policy. 2018;11:263–71. Published 2018 Dec 7. https://doi.org/10.2147/RMHP.S156404.
21. Rosekind MR, Smith RM, Miller DL, Co EL, Gregory KB, Webbon LL, Gander PH, Lebacqz JV. Alertness management: strategic naps in operational settings. J Sleep Res. 1995;4(S2):62–6. https://doi.org/10.1111/j.1365-2869.1995.tb00229.x.
22. Rampling CM, Gupta CC, Shriane AE, Ferguson SA, Rigney G, Vincent GE. Does knowledge of sleep hygiene recommendations match behaviour in Australian shift workers? A cross-sectional study. BMJ Open. 2022;12(7):e059677. Published 2022 Jul 6. https://doi.org/10.1136/bmjopen-2021-059677.
23. Smith JL, Allen JW, Haack CI, et al. Impact of app-delivered mindfulness meditation on functional connectivity, mental health, and sleep disturbances among physician assistant students: randomized, wait-list controlled pilot study. JMIR Form Res. 2021;5(10):e24208. Published 2021 Oct 19. https://doi.org/10.2196/24208.
24. Fang Y, Forger DB, Frank E, Sen S, Goldstein C. Day-to-day variability in sleep parameters and depression risk: a prospective cohort study of training physicians. NPJ Digit Med. 2021;4(1):28. Published 2021 Feb 18. https://doi.org/10.1038/s41746-021-00400-z.

Chapter 40
Nutrition and Exercise: Maintaining a Healthy Lifestyle in Surgery Residency

Joseph Sciacca

Introduction

The unpredictable hours of surgical residency can be challenging for a surgical resident, especially when it comes to diet, nutrition, and exercise. In this chapter, I share a personal take on how to maintain your health and nutrition goals. I hope this inspires those reading to place more focus on their nutrition and how it relates to their health.

Long hours. Stress. Responsibility overload.
And now, some unsolicited nutrition advice.

Maintaining pre-residency life is a significant challenge for most surgical residents. Diet and nutrition become an often-overlooked aspect of a resident's life, and it is typically one of the easiest habits to neglect. Between quick cafeteria trips on night shift, energy drinks, and calorie-dense specialty coffees, the overall health of a resident can rapidly deteriorate. With the variability of a surgeon's schedule, it is easy to look for fast and convenient options.

Before residency, I took pride in grocery shopping, cooking, and eating healthy. I have kept my diet aligned with my nutrition and fitness goals. I continue to shop for groceries and prepare my meals throughout the week. Continuing these habits allows me to be prepared for the nights when I leave work late. Instead of scurrying to the nearest drive-through, I have healthy food waiting at home. This lifestyle requires significant determination, but the benefits of increased energy, cognitive clarity, and body image are worthwhile.

J. Sciacca (✉)
Christiana Care Health System, Newark, DE, USA
e-mail: joseph.sciacca@christianacare.org

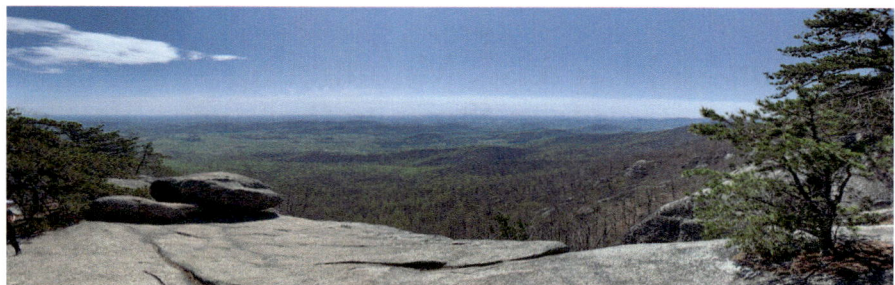

Fig. 40.1 Here is a beautiful panoramic view from near the top of Old Rag Mountain, Shenandoah National Park, in Virginia!

Grocery shopping can be time consuming and a barrier to achieving nutritional goals. Thankfully, the movement toward app-based grocery delivery allows the busy surgery resident to obtain healthy food without wasting the limited precious time they have away from work. By whichever means I obtain my food, I stick to a trio of lean meat, steamed vegetables, and a healthy source of carbohydrates. These choices work best for me, as they enable me to enjoy those "cheat meals" that will not add to an accumulation of frequent unhealthy meals. On a sidenote, if you are interested in utilizing companies that prepare meals for you, make sure that you read the nutritional content. Sodium, carbohydrates, and fats can be well hidden, making those meals work against your goals.

My last piece of nutrition advice comes from personal preference and shared knowledge. Calories come in many forms, and the sneakiest of them all are liquids. I am referring to soda, sugary energy drinks, and complicated coffee shop orders. The human body does not experience the same satiety from an 800-calorie beverage as it does from a well-balanced meal of the same number of calories. The result is overeating, higher calorie consumption, and dreaded weight gain. I urge all residents to do their best in curbing their intake. Moderation is key.

In closing, I would like to encourage an active lifestyle (Fig. 40.1). With the unpredictable hours and constant shift changes, exercising can disappear for residents. Keeping things simple, short outdoor walks, taking the stairs at work, purchasing small pieces of exercise equipment, or taking advantage of a hospital gym can help maximize efficiency. Fitness trackers, new exercise clothes, and music can be extraordinary motivators. Do what you can throughout the course of the day to stay active.

Pearls

Nutrition is about mindset and execution. In the end, I will leave you with this:

- It is important to enjoy your life, so do (and eat) what makes YOU happy.
- As physicians, we serve as role models of health to our patients.
- Moderation is key!

Chapter 41
Self-Care: When and How

Madison Harris and Arielle Brackett

Introduction

For all the hype and social media attention, self-care for the surgical resident continues to seem both illusive and daunting. While the touted all-inclusive resort weekend getaways or 12-step skin care routines may not be feasible for the average resident, the truth is that self-care encompasses any conscious act a person takes to promote their physical, mental, and emotional health. Read on for ideas to make self-care work for you.

While we do not claim to be experts, nor do we intend to use this space to expound the benefits of self-care (which are many), we do think that it is important to acknowledge the difference that a small investment into yourself can have on personal health and interactions with the people and world around you. As residents, we spend much of our time taking care of others, frequently putting our personal needs aside to address the needs of our patients. Though this is commended in some circles and viewed as a necessary "part of the job," the downstream effects can include hastened burnout, career dissatisfaction, depression, and anxiety. Redirecting a small fraction of your time to the activities and practices that "fill your cup" will not only keep you healthy but also enable you to be an even better physician, colleague, and teammate.

A key step is adopting the mental framework that self-care is not a luxury or another task on your never-ending to-do list, but a practice that should be prioritized for your physical, mental, and emotional well-being. Sometimes, it can be as simple as letting yourself get eight plus hours of sleep or bypassing the Chick-fil-A on your way home for something you prepare yourself. Another realization that has been

M. Harris (✉) · A. Brackett
Christiana Care Health System, Newark, DE, USA
e-mail: madison.harris@christianacare.org; arielle.brackett@christianacare.org

A. Ratnasekera et al. (eds.), *General Surgery Residency Survival Guide*,
https://doi.org/10.1007/978-3-031-25617-2_41

meaningful for us personally is that there are no right or wrong ways to practice self-care. For example, Madison cares for herself by meal-prepping, meditating, and religiously performing her nighttime skin care routine. Arielle, on the other hand, frequently skips face-washing but becomes a cranky monster if she does not have time for a workout.

Self-reflection is paramount to your self-care practice. If you feel physically run down after a long day of cases, triaging consults, or managing patients on the floor, and need a break from those fluorescent hospital lights, then maybe a short walk outside after work to get fresh air and vitamin D is the answer. If you feel mentally overstimulated and need some mind-numbing reality TV, queue up *Love Island* for a break. If you feel emotionally exhausted and need to decompress, perhaps you call or get together with a family member, close friend, or co-resident to unpack the day's events or catch up on something completely unrelated. Perhaps you feel totally fine at work, but what truly brings you joy is playing competitive soccer, sketching, gardening, or spending time with loved ones (Fig. 41.1). Carve out time to cultivate these interests and hobbies and connect with the people who matter most—you will thank yourself later!

Okay, we will admit that last point is much easier said than done. But despite the perceived difficulty, it is important to remember that we are each accountable for our own well-being; only you know how to best take care of you. Again, self-care will not look the same for everyone, and your self-care will not look the same every day—this is okay. But we encourage you to continue to find ways to show up for yourself—you are worth it.

Fig. 41.1 Madison's plot at her local community garden

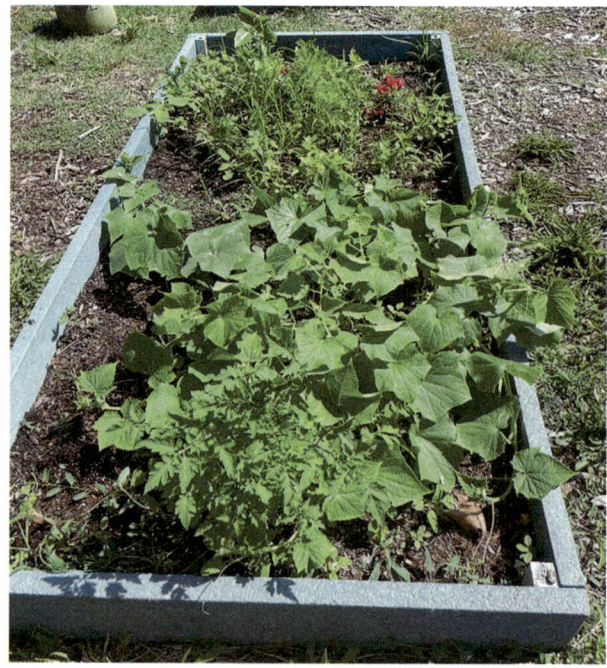

Pearls
- Self-care is not a luxury but a practice that should be prioritized for your physical, mental, and emotional well-being.
- Self-reflection is paramount to meaningful self-care.
- We are each accountable for our own well-being.

Chapter 42
Stress Management and Dealing with Burnout

Sirivan Seng

Identifying Stress and Burnout

Surgical residency is, without a doubt, a stressful time. Television often glamorizes residency training; however, the reality is a far cry from what the public perceive it to be. The stress is often overwhelming and can lead to burnout. It can lead to debilitating anxiety, decreased energy, clinical depression, substance abuse, high-risk behavior, or even suicidal ideation [1]. In fact, a national survey conducted after an annual In-Training Examination in 2018 reported that 38.5% surgical residents reported having weekly burnout symptoms and 4.5% had suicidal thoughts during the past year [2].

So how does one identify stress? This can be extremely difficult in the busy everyday life as a surgical resident. Some symptoms of stress can manifest in the obvious form of increased heart rate, chest pain, body aches, grinding your teeth, clenching your jaw, waking up with a sore jaw, shortness of breath, changes in bowel habits, changes in weight, changes in eating habits, or decreased libido. Other symptoms that may be more difficult to identify are being more emotional, decreased concentration, decreased memory, or turning to alcohol or other substances for relief. It is important to identify these symptoms should you be experiencing them yourself or if you see them in your colleagues.

S. Seng (✉)
Crozer Chester Medical Center, Upland, PA, USA
e-mail: sirivan.seng@crozer.org

Methods of Management

You cannot calm the storm, so stop trying. What you can do is calm yourself, the storm will pass.—Timber Hawkeye

It is okay if you recognize that you may be overworked and overwhelmed. The stress of surgical residency is not something that one can be prepared for, but is rather managed day by day by building coping skills. Medicine is constantly advancing, and the job of a surgical resident has changed drastically over the past hundreds of years. Not only must you have the medical knowledge, but you must also perform open, laparoscopic, and robotic surgery; complete administrative paperwork; participate in research; and possibly plan to compete for fellowships, all the while attempting to maintain a social life, keep up with friends and family, pay your bills, and sleep.

When you recognize that you are stressed or burnt out, it is vital that you verbalize it. There are many people around you that you can tell. This can include trusted colleagues—who can also sometimes commiserate with you—a mentor, your program director, or even a family member or friend. The first step is to acknowledge that there is an issue. From that point, there are many options. Sometimes, taking a few personal days to sit at home and do nothing, spending time with family, going on a vacation, taking a research year, speaking with a counselor, or even practicing yoga or mindfulness can help alleviate the stress. One institution provided their surgical interns with formal resilience training throughout their first year and found that there was a decreased risk of depression, suicidal ideation, burnout, and stress [3]. Because the field of medicine is a roller coaster of emotions even after residency, it is important that you build the coping skills to lift yourself out of those down moments and find ways to get back in the game. The only way to truly provide the best care for your patients is to make sure that you take care of yourself first.

Pearls
- Residency inherently is full of stressors. It is important to learn coping skills to succeed.
- Prioritize activities that make you happy, even the small things. They will keep you sane in the long run.
- Be on the lookout for your colleagues as well as yourself for signs of burnout.

References

1. Lebares CC, Guvva EV, Ascher NL, O'Sullivan PS, Harris HW, Epel ES. Burnout and stress among US surgery residents: psychological distress and resilience. J Am Coll Surg. 2018;226(1):80–90. https://doi.org/10.1016/j.jamcollsurg.2017.10.010.
2. Hu YY, Ellis RJ, Hewitt DB, Yang AD, Cheung EO, Moskowitz JT, Potts JR 3rd, Buyske J, Hoyt DB, Nasca TJ, Bilimoria KY. Discrimination, abuse, harassment, and burnout in surgical residency training. N Engl J Med. 2019;381(18):1741–52. https://doi.org/10.1056/NEJMsa1903759.
3. Lebares CC, Hershberger AO, Guvva EV, Desai A, Mitchell J, Shen W, Reilly LM, Delucchi KL, O'Sullivan PS, Ascher NL, Harris HW. Feasibility of formal mindfulness-based stress-resilience training among surgery interns: a randomized clinical trial. JAMA Surg. 2018;153(10):e182734. https://doi.org/10.1001/jamasurg.2018.2734.

Chapter 43
What to Do on Vacation

Madison Harris and Arielle Brackett

Introduction

Time away from work seems like a simple topic to discuss, but there is much to consider with a limited window outside of the hospital. The vacations that we eagerly anticipate for months pass by quickly, leaving us wistful and hungry for the next one. Below are our tips for making the most of your time off.

First, think about what kind of vacation you want and/or need. As our time off is limited, there can be a lot of pressure to do something *exciting* or, even worse, *productive*. Some self-reflection can go a long way here: For instance, are you looking to slow down and relax, or recharge with an adventure to some new place? Do you need to spend time alone, or are you longing to reconnect with family and friends? There is no right or wrong answer here, and there should be absolutely no guilt in the decisions you make—the most important thing is that you are honest with yourself and your needs. Personally, we have a couple of different approaches: Madison will try to do a little bit of everything with her week off, while Arielle tries to work in a variety of activities throughout the course of the year (e.g., 1 week off for an adventure, the next week off for friends and family). Again, there is no right answer, just the answer that works best for you.

Planning a vacation can be an intimidating task. It is time consuming and often involves research, especially if you are flying or using public transit. Try to start preparing early and chip away at tasks over the preceding weeks to months. If traveling with partners, assign tasks such as booking flights and hotels and scheduling activities. Do not feel pressured to have an itinerary for each day—sometimes, the

M. Harris (✉) · A. Brackett
Christiana Care Health System, Newark, DE, USA
e-mail: madison.harris@christianacare.org; arielle.brackett@christianacare.org

© The Author(s), under exclusive license to Springer Nature Switzerland AG 2023
A. Ratnasekera et al. (eds.), *General Surgery Residency Survival Guide*,
https://doi.org/10.1007/978-3-031-25617-2_43

best journeys are not planned at all. One of our biggest personal challenges in residency is the grossly undervalued time for family. Vacations are the holy grail of uninterrupted time with loved ones. Once you know your schedule, share your vacation blocks with your family and friends ahead of time to allow for overlapping breaks.

Next, consider how much time off is allotted. Does your program allow 2-week vacations, 1-week vacations, or a combination of both? Will you have the preceding weekend off, transforming a 1-week vacation into a *blessed* 9 days? If this is not something that is guaranteed, it may be worth exploring the possibility of swapping a weekend with a co-resident—especially if you are planning to travel domestically or internationally. It is also important to consider your financial means. Between student loans, home/car payments, and other financial obligations, vacations are sometimes a luxury we cannot afford. Here, setting a realistic budget can be your best friend. You may decide that one, or all, of your weeks off will be a staycation—and that is 100% okay! If you go this route, try not to skimp on the planning. Like we said, you do not need to have an itinerary for each day, but this can be a great opportunity to explore the surrounding area through a new lens.

Once you are actually on your vacation, *unplug and disconnect*. If checking your email is stressful for you—*do not do it*. We are big fans of out-of-office replies. More important than removing yourself from work is taking the time to enjoy and appreciate the world outside the hospital. Allow yourself to be immersed in the experience and reconnect with the activities and people that remind you that you are more than just a surgery resident. When you have those moments which allow you to reconnect with your passions and humanity, hold on to them! Arielle is a big fan of documenting—be it through journaling, photos, or even Instagram stories: anything that can help bring you back to those moments where you feel most like you (Figs. 43.1 and 43.2). Revisiting these memories can help spark joy once you are back on the wards.

"Sunday Scaries" are no joke, and transitioning back to work can be a challenge. While we personally have not found a way to avoid the post-vacation slump (and exhaustion that can come with it), we will share a couple of things that help us make it through. Try to clean before you leave so you come back to a sparkling house and less mess. Unpack before you go back to work, or that suitcase will sit in the corner of your room for an intolerable amount of time. Plan a fun activity during your first week and/or weekend back to have something to look forward to; this can be as small as a dinner with co-residents or seeing that movie you have been meaning to catch. Or maybe, it is sitting down and planning out your next vacation—cheers!

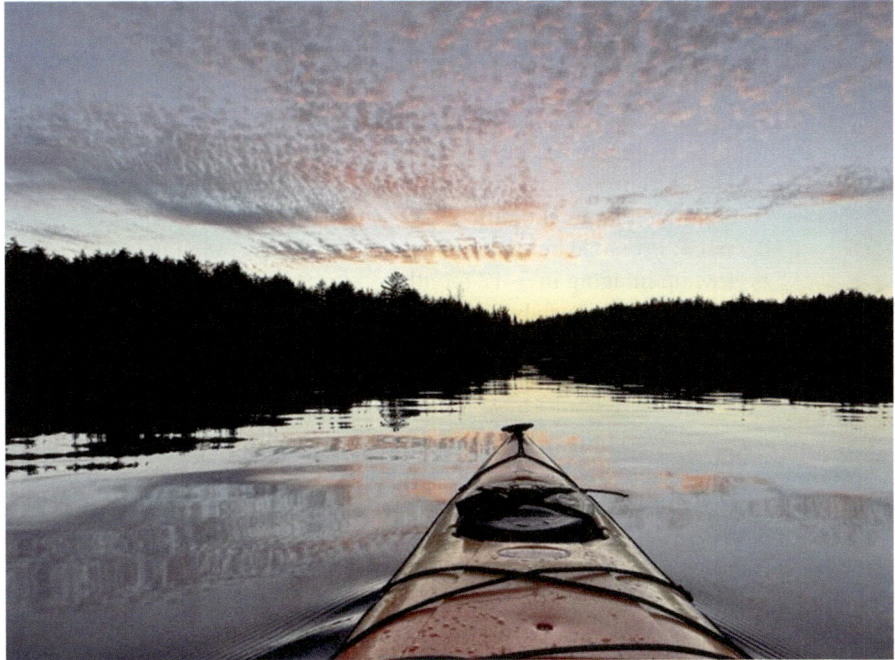

Fig. 43.1 Sunset paddle on Saranac Lake, NY—October 2021

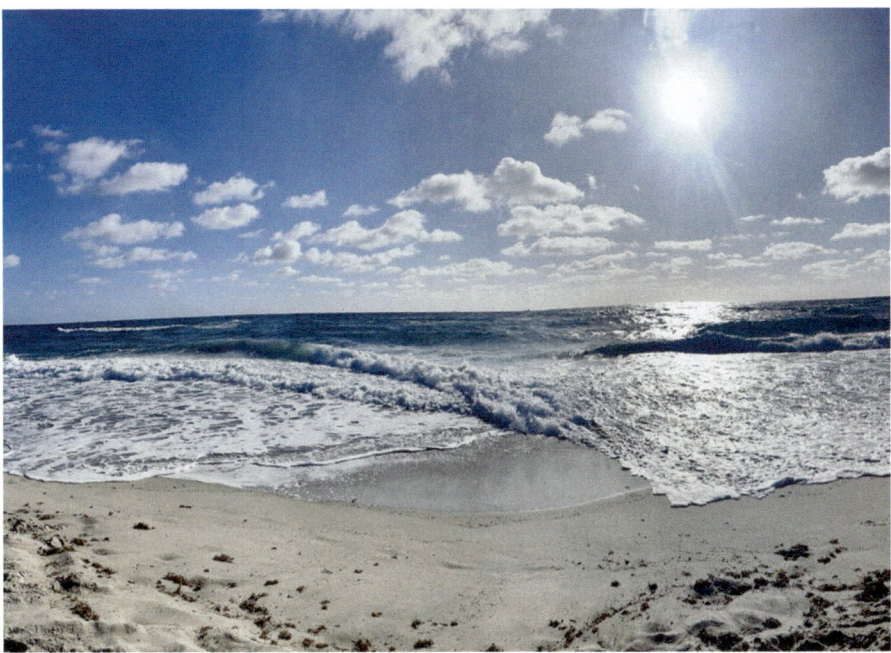

Fig. 43.2 Morning walk in Delray Beach, FL—February 2022

Pearls
- Be honest about the type of vacation you want and need.
- It is never too early to start planning your next trip.
- Unpack your suitcase before you go back to work.

Chapter 44
Making Time for Hobbies

Madison Harris

Introduction

Think of activities you do regularly in your leisure time that bring you pleasure. These are your hobbies. Whether it be carving out time for friends and family, exercising, or preparing a home-cooked meal, making time for the things that reliably bring you joy will make residency much more manageable. I may not be an expert, but I have first-hand experience in making little joys a big part of my life.

Ask any surgery resident to list their hobbies and one will undoubtedly be "operating." When thinking of my hobbies, my mind races as if filling out a resumé of professionally acceptable activities. The reality is that my hobbies are simple: cooking, catching up on TV, gardening, and walking. Nothing noble, nothing outrageous, just things I truly enjoy when my schedule allows.

How do we find time for the things we love when working 80 h a week? I will be the first to admit that it is no simple feat. Making room for my hobbies takes away time from other activities: studying, sleeping, and even showering. But the joy they bring me is well worth the extra day of greasy hair and darker circles under my eyes. If you have activities that you enjoy before residency, try to stay true to them for the five-plus-year journey. It is easy to lose sight of things that do not involve work and sleep during residency. Priorities change and your hobbies may change too, but find activities that give you a sense of relief and do not feel like an obligation.

While residency can be all-consuming, keep in mind that it is just one part of your life. One of my hobbies is maintaining close relationships with friends from college and medical school. Planning scheduled Zoom calls or weekend visits is a great way for me to unwind. You can also find ways to get involved in your new

M. Harris (✉)
Christiana Care Health System, Newark, DE, USA
e-mail: madison.harris@christianacare.org

community. For example, growing vegetables at my local community garden plot gives me a sense of purpose and keeps me healthy with fresh produce (a win-win situation!) (Fig. 44.1). Even local farmers' markets and walking trails can become part of your routine. I always tweak the things most important to me to make them work in my schedule, such as keeping plants in my apartment year-round and using my Peloton when it is too cold (or I am too lazy) to walk outside. Wrapping up the day with a home-cooked meal or freshly baked cookie provides me with consistent happiness (Fig. 44.2).

Fig. 44.1 My community garden plot

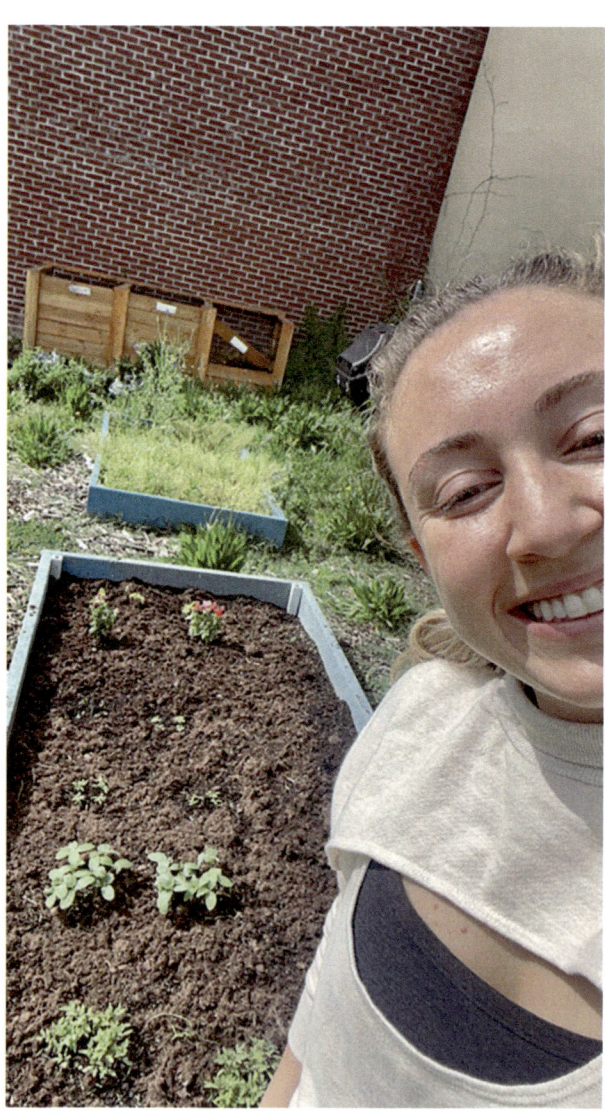

Fig. 44.2 Home-baked
chocolate chip cookies

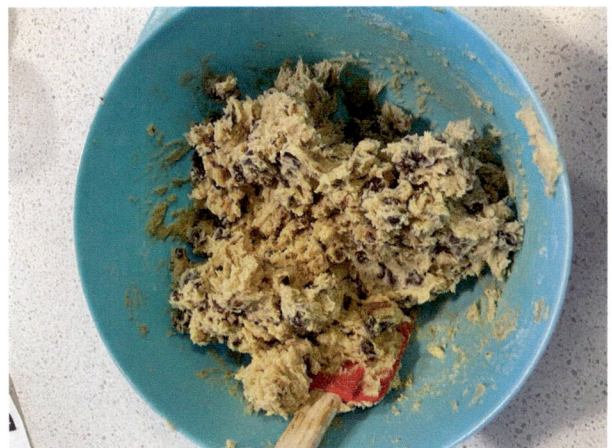

I must confess that not all of my passions can be enmeshed into a busy surgical schedule. I save leisurely reading and soaking up the sun for dedicated vacation time (see chapter on *Vacations*). With that being said, it is essential to maintain the restorative pursuits that make you whole (also see chapter on *Self-care*). Preserve your friendships, make time for family, and fine-tune your hobbies to fit into a life where surgery will always be a dominating hobby.

Pearls
- Make time for the things that reliably bring you joy.
- Find activities that give you a sense of relief and do not feel like an obligation.
- Preserve your friendships and make time for family.

Chapter 45
Illness and Injury During Residency

Bradford Bormann

The first day back from vacation is demoralizing, especially when you got married over the break. I was staring into the abyssal EMR in our call room, a gentle tickle in my overworked larynx and a gleaming ring on my finger, wishing the glorious reprieve could have lasted a bit longer. My phone buzzes, my sister is calling, forgoing the casual text in a foreboding sign that something was amiss.

"What's up?" I answer.

"Do you have a minute?" She asks, her voice scratchy and soft. "I took a rapid test …" was all she had to say.

Suddenly the tickle in my throat felt more sinister and my surgical mask wore paper-thin. In a whir I was home on the couch, COVID positive, ironically getting the reprieve I had been hoping for and riddled with guilt for it.

Fact: Illness and injury will happen during residency. Here are some insights for when it happens to you:

Do not look a gift horse in the mouth. In other words, take the break as the opportunity to heal that it is meant to be, without judging the time as unmerited. Residency is an unrelenting effort to improve oneself, but in this instance, it is best to truly unplug, detach, and heal. Do not feel guilt for this; it is quite literally your job to "get better" during this time.

If you have a communicable disease, you owe it to your patients to stay home. Do no harm. Patients are lying on their backs in bed, hoping that your actions and orders will help them to heal. Do not halt their progress by dumping pathogens onto them during morning rounds.

B. Bormann (✉)
Christiana Care Health System, Newark, DE, USA
e-mail: bradford.bormann@christianacare.org

© The Author(s), under exclusive license to Springer Nature
Switzerland AG 2023
A. Ratnasekera et al. (eds.), *General Surgery Residency Survival Guide*,
https://doi.org/10.1007/978-3-031-25617-2_45

Similarly, patients deserve the best care you can offer. If you have an injury which compromises the care you offer (like a surgeon with a hairline humeral fracture—true story), let another colleague step in. The patient will understand and appreciate your self-awareness.

You will likely feel guilty. At baseline, the resident workforce is stretched thin to the point of becoming transparent. Losing a healthy worker means everyone else has to stretch that much further to accommodate. Sitting at home and unable to contribute may make you feel embarrassed and unworthy, maybe even subject to the private and frustrated comments of colleagues having to cover. The bottom line is that at some point, everyone will be sidelined. You will get to do this for someone else. Allow your teammates to cover for you and give yourself grace, because at some point, you will do the same for them while hoping that they rest and come back in full strength.

Find a way to improve and contribute. If you begin to feel well enough and you still have some mandatory time away from work, do a little extra reading, work on a project, or get administrative tasks done. Even 20 min of productivity may help you lay your head at night without being dogged by the sentiment that "I wasted today."

Pearls
- It is important to realize that you must have a sense of well-being to be able to take care of patients.
- In the event of sickness or injury, take the time to recover while being productive and completing administrative tasks.

Chapter 46
Dealing with a Pandemic

Sirivan Seng

COVID-19 and Pandemonium

The COVID-19 pandemic brought about many changes to everyday life. Hospitals were overwhelmed with too many patients, too little staff, and dwindling resources. As a result, elective cases were canceled across the United States in an attempt to conserve resources and decrease exposure.

The pandemic also greatly affected surgical training. Resident lectures and grand rounds were transitioned into remote virtual learning [1]. Some surgical residents were pulled into medical intensive care units to care for patients with which they may not have had prior experience [2]. Since elective cases were canceled, operative volume significantly decreased. Many attendings and residents were diagnosed with or exposed to COVID-19, mandating weeks of quarantine and loss of work hours. In our institution, we transitioned to an "on-call" system, where only call residents were present in the hospital to minimize exposure and therefore maintain the resident workforce to enhance coverage. Sometimes, this could be Q3 call with a skeleton crew in the hospital to take care of patients at all times, which meant that you were responsible for all patients on all services at the time. Such changes placed a significant strain on the medical education system. In a survey of surgical residents, one study found that the majority of residents were only performing 1–3 cases a week during the height of the pandemic. However, residents had ample more opportunities to study and perform research [3].

S. Seng (✉)
Crozer Chester Medical Center, Upland, PA, USA
e-mail: sirivan.seng@crozer.org

A. Ratnasekera et al. (eds.), *General Surgery Residency Survival Guide*,
https://doi.org/10.1007/978-3-031-25617-2_46

193

Survival Skills for Pandemonium While in Residency

One of the most important tools in the medical professional's toolbox, and particularly a surgical resident's, is adaptability. A surgical resident often transitions from location to location at different hospitals and must adapt quickly to different work environments to facilitate good patient care. We have to remain adaptable in different clinical situations such as codes or caring for very sick patients. Remaining flexible in these highly stressful situations will help you succeed with whatever future changes may arise.

In order to compensate for the lack of surgical cases and operative time, take the initiative to take part in training modules that may be available to you. When there is downtime, dive into a surgical textbook or atlas. Additionally, many surgical societies such as the American College of Surgeons (ACS) and the Society of American Gastrointestinal and Endoscopic Surgeons (SAGES) have instructional videos on how to perform surgeries and give helpful tips on how to be the most efficient at your craft. During the few times you have the opportunity to put those skills into use, you will be well read and ready. It is important to focus on the things that you can do rather than dwell on what could have been.

This is also a great time to complete those research projects that had taken a back burner. Revisit your things-to-do list, catch up on administrative tasks, and complete case logging. Finally, this could be the time to spend with your family and friends.

Despite these changes, surgical residents learned many important lessons of pandemic management, disease containment, and critical care management of very sick COVID-19 patients, and it is likely (and perhaps hopefully) a once-in-a-lifetime opportunity.

Pearls
- Flexibility and adaptability are key to making it through a pandemic.
- Time away from the hospital could be utilized to catch up on research, administrative duties, or family responsibilities.

References

1. Wise CE, Bereknyei Merrell S, Sasnal M, Forrester JD, Hawn MT, Lau JN, Lin DT, Schmiederer IS, Spain DA, Nassar AK, Knowlton LM. COVID-19 impact on surgical resident education and coping. J Surg Res. 2021;264:534–43. https://doi.org/10.1016/j.jss.2021.01.017. Epub 2021 Feb 11
2. Samuel N. Surgical residents at the forefront of the COVID-19 pandemic: perspectives on redeployment. Ann Surg. 2021;274(5):e383–4. https://doi.org/10.1097/SLA.0000000000004991.
3. Aziz H, James T, Remulla D, Sher L, Genyk Y, Sullivan ME, Sheikh MR. Effect of COVID-19 on surgical training across the United States: a national survey of general surgery residents. J Surg Educ. 2021;78(2):431–9. https://doi.org/10.1016/j.jsurg.2020.07.037. Epub 2020 Jul 30

Chapter 47
How to Navigate a Brand-New Residency Program

Ammar Humayun

Introduction

Starting at a new residency program can sound like the scariest thing out there (aside from Florida alligators outside your doorstep). There are lots of *challenges* associated with a new residency program. These challenges can be used to become your strengths, not only during residency, but also after its completion.

One of the challenges of being in a new residency program can be insecurity. New residency programs typically have a probationary period in which they are "under a microscope" by the ACGME to ensure that all requirements and educational commitments are being fulfilled. You may feel insecure about the program, unsure of what type of education it has to offer you, and uncertain of what challenges you will face after you graduate. It may seem like you are taking a huge leap into an unknown dark hole.

What Does This Mean for You?

This means that the program will try very hard to make sure that you are getting the appropriate training; the appropriate procedures (if you are in an interventional field); the appropriate number of hours off; and the rest of the typical requirements (i.e., educational stipend, meal allowance, call rooms).

A. Humayun (✉)
Crozer Medical Center, Upland, PA, USA
e-mail: ammar.humayun@crozer.org

This also means that you have to understand that there may be some hurdles and growing pains. There may be days when the ideal call schedule is not possible or you may have to fill in more if one of your colleagues get sick, etc. *All this shall pass with time.* When I started my general surgery residency, we were in every third night call (and occasionally every other night call) and did not have a single 2-day weekend off. It was extremely tough; the COVID pandemic hit, which did not help; but now we look back at it and think to ourselves that the experience has only taught us a significant amount about ourselves and made us extremely resilient and prepared for the worst-case scenario (Figs. 47.1 and 47.2).

One of the biggest advantages to being in a new residency program is that there is room for growth and leadership. You have the opportunity to be at the forefront of your residency; to develop the program from the ground-up; to contribute your values and ideas to how the program can be better; and to shape it for yourself and future residents to come. When I started residency, we would have meetings about which rotations we should cover, call schedules, plans for resident-retreats, and interdepartmental issues. All these meetings translated in real time to practical solutions and improvements in the program. It is very satisfying to see your discussions being converted to practical changes in your program. This also helps you develop your leadership skills to engage and lead a group of residents to make changes for the better (Fig. 47.3).

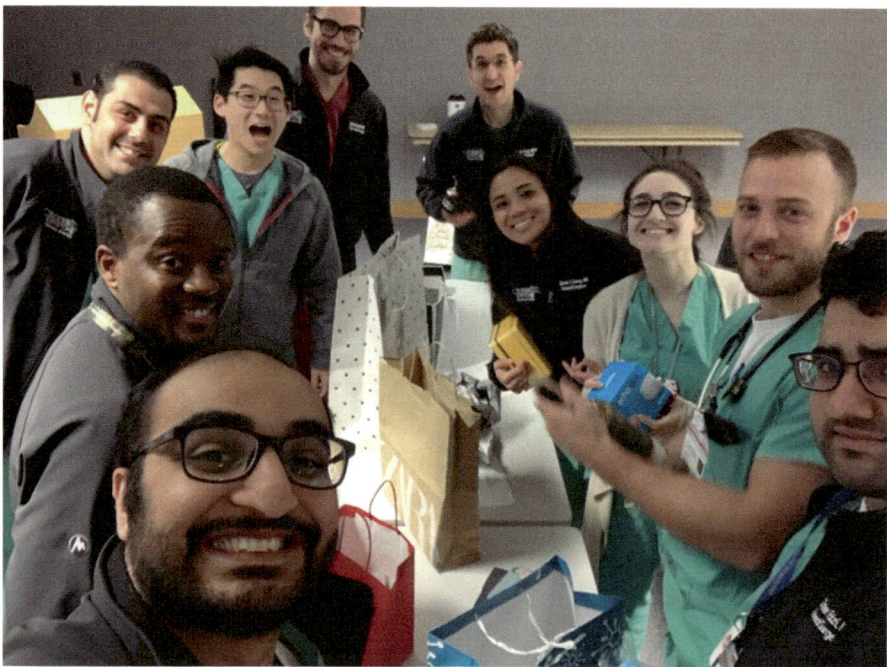

Fig. 47.1 Founding Fathers/Mothers of Our Residency at Crozer Medical Center sharing gifts during Secret Santa

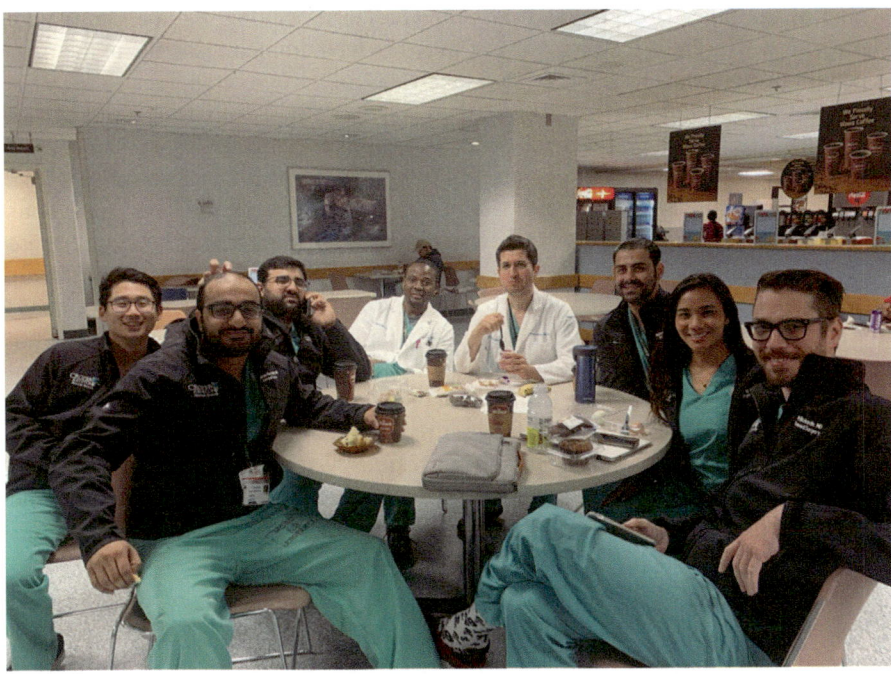

Fig. 47.2 Some of the original residents in our brand-new program

Fig. 47.3 I am taking lead
in ICU teaching rounds

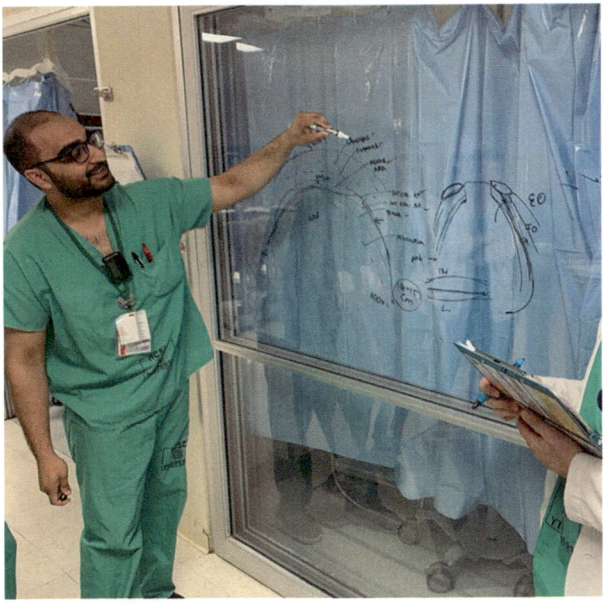

One of the other strengths and possible challenges can be the attendings with whom you work. The attendings may or may not have trained residents in the past. Depending on their experience, it may take time for certain attendings to increase their level of comfort and trust with the residents. This is ok! It is important to understand that. The attendings you work with will be excited to have residents and to pass on the torch of knowledge; this will be a great experience for you (Fig. 47.4).

Not only will the attendings with whom you work be grateful to have continuous interactions with residents they are training, but also the hospital at large will share the same sentiments. These providers are no longer required to work with people who occasionally come from outside institutes or who may show their face every now and then and then never be seen again. You are now part of the hospital. You are part of the group of physicians that develop rapport with the nursing staff, operating room staff, X-ray technicians, ER staff, and other consultants. Any one of these may be your referral base one day, or even your patient! (See Fig. 47.5.)

The relationships you make during your residency will carry on even after your residency. You will meet other residents, attendings, and staff from all pathways and all walks of life. When we started residency, we had many preliminary residents from all over the country coming with their own experiences and backgrounds.

Fig. 47.4 Operating with one of my favorite trauma attendings

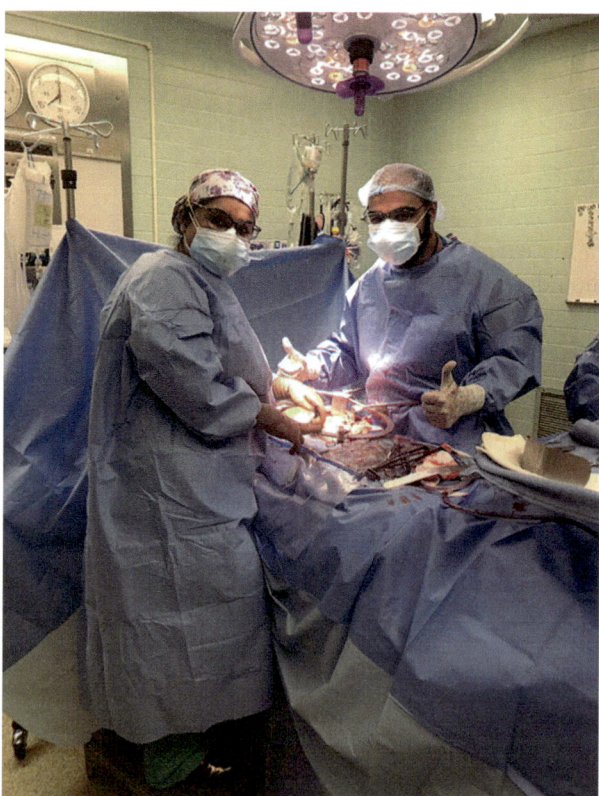

Fig. 47.5 Another night in the ICU

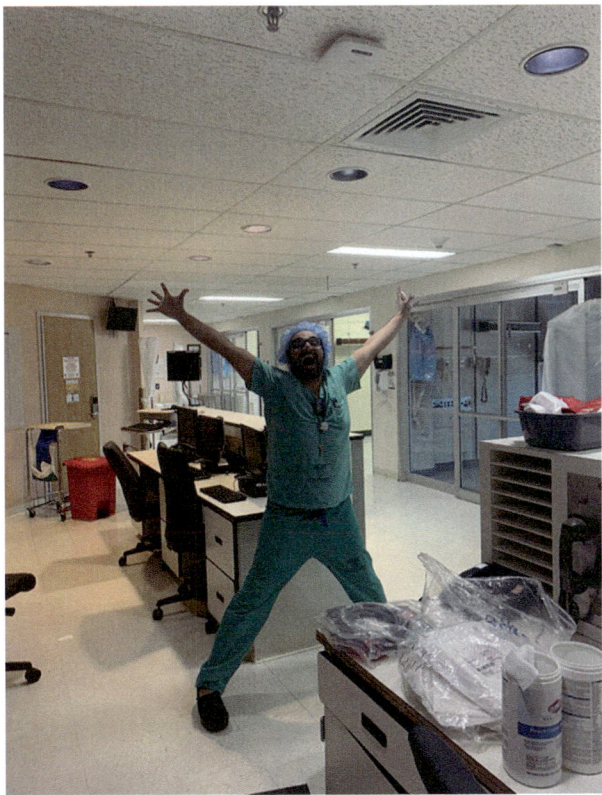

Initially, this may appear to be a challenge, but with good collegiality and understanding, this can easily be transformed into a strength of a program. The bonds and experience you share with these residents who will go through the same experience as you are unique.

Pearls
- It is by no means going to be a walk in the park—be prepared to face challenges, yet *embrace* these challenges to become your strengths.
- You will have many people vouching for you, including your residency attendings, your program director, your colleagues, and most importantly the ACGME—they all want to see YOU succeed.
- Use the opportunity to become a leader. A new residency program will give you leadership traits and opportunities that many other well-established programs may not.

Chapter 48
Imposter Syndrome During Surgical Training

Michael Johns

Introduction

The origin of the term *imposter syndrome* is attributed to American psychologists, Pauline Clance and Suzanne Imes [1]. Their original study involved high-achieving women, who earned PhDs, who were respected in their fields, or were students recognized for their academic excellence. Clance and Imes found that some women did not experience an internal sense of success, despite "their earned degrees, scholastic honors, high achievement on standardized tests, praise, and professional recognition" [1].

Since that time, imposter syndrome has been studied in many fields, including medicine, humanities, sciences, economics, and philosophy. While the initial discussion focused on women, there is evidence that many men feel similarly, showing even greater anxiety than women after receiving negative feedback and under conditions of high accountability [2].

From the psychology literature, Leary et al. described the three key attributes central to imposter syndrome: the sense of being a fraud, fear of being discovered, and difficulty internalizing success [3].

There are many scoring systems used to delineate the severity of imposter syndrome including the Clance Impostor Phenomenon Survey (CIPS), Harvey Imposter Scale, Perceived Fraudulence Scale, and Leary Impostor Scale [4]. Common signs of imposter syndrome include:

- Fear of not being good enough for a job/task
- Feeling inauthentic and deceptive

M. Johns (✉)
Fellow, Colorectal Surgery, Brown University, Providence, RI, USA

© The Author(s), under exclusive license to Springer Nature Switzerland AG 2023
A. Ratnasekera et al. (eds.), *General Surgery Residency Survival Guide*,
https://doi.org/10.1007/978-3-031-25617-2_48

- Doubting your ability to be successful
- Fear of some loss (income, employment, relationships)
- Fear of failure
- Feeling of not belonging to current role

While the true incidence of imposter syndrome amongst medical professionals is not known, it is pervasive throughout many specialties. A recent study at 6-ACGME-accredited general surgery programs showed that 98.9% of surgical residents who responded by filling out the CIPS scored moderate, significant, or intense levels of imposter syndrome and only 2.1% exhibited mild levels or no symptoms [5]. Interestingly, there was no difference in CIPS scores when comparing for sex ($p = 0.69$), age ($p = 0.46$), race ($p = 0.07$), USMLE scores ($p = 0.34$), ABSITE scores ($p = 0.17$), or PGY level ($p = 0.72$). The results highlight the fact that imposter syndrome is widely variable and affects many surgical trainees, not one particular group [5].

Tips for Managing Imposter Syndrome

It is important not to "bottle up" your feelings. Talk to someone who will support you, who can recognize the enormous amount of work you have accomplished to get to this point. Ask a close friend for an honest viewpoint. It is important to recognize feelings of imposter syndrome and work to validate yourself before it leads to panic attacks or anxiety. To tackle imposter syndrome, focus on healthy self-talk, identify your successes, and ground your mental state. Here are some suggestions:

- Make a list—spell out your accomplishments to date, and revisit. Ask yourself is there anything that makes you *less* qualified than anyone else?
- Take time for enjoyable activities—take a step back and allow your mental health to recover and do some physical activity to remove any anxiety/angst.
- Take breaks from social media—this can lead to unfair and harmful comparisons.

Lastly, it is important to realize that you can harness some feelings of imposter syndrome to work in your favor. If maintained at a low level, using these feelings can push you to set a reading schedule during residency, become more involved with research projects, and ensure that you will achieve and recognize your successes.

Pearls
- Imposter syndrome can affect all surgical trainees, regardless of sex, clinical performance, test scores, race, or age.
- Utilizing a good network, focusing on your own achievements and goals, and reminding yourself of your accomplishments to date can help you keep a good perspective about your journey.
- In certain cases, these feelings of imposter syndrome can motivate you to study, publish more research, and work harder, which can pay dividends in the future.

References

1. Clance PR, Imes SA. The imposter phenomenon in high achieving women: dynamics and therapeutic intervention. Psychol Psychother. 1978;15:241–7.
2. Badawy RL, Gazdag BA, Bentley JR, Brouer RL. Are all impostors created equal? Exploring gender differences in the impostor phenomenon-performance link. Pers Individ Differ. 2018;131:156–63.
3. Leary MR, Patton KM, Orlando AE, Wagoner Funk W. The impostor phenomenon: self-perceptions, reflected appraisals, and interpersonal strategies. J Pers. 2000;68(4):725–56.
4. Mak KKL, Kleitman S, Abbott MJ. Impostor phenomenon measurement scales: a systematic review. Front Psychol. 2019;10:671.
5. Bhama AR, Ritz EM, Anand RJ, Auyang ED, Lipman J, Greenberg JA, Kapadia MR. Imposter syndrome in surgical trainees: Clance imposter phenomenon scale assessment in general surgery residents. J Am Coll Surg. 2021;233(5):633–8.

Chapter 49
Conclusion

Sirivan Seng

Residency can be one of the most trying times of your life. There is nothing more revealing about your own personality than when you are put into a pressure cooker with a whole hospital filled with strangers. You certainly cannot control everything that happens during these years, but your flexibility, adaptability, and resilience will be your biggest asset. Time will fly by faster than you think. Suddenly, the countdown that you have on your calendar, whether it be physical or mental, will drop down from over 1800 days to 100 days, before you can even blink. There is a lot sacrificed on the journey to becoming a surgeon, but the end is filled with much reward.

The authors of this book wish you the best of luck during these next few years. Cherish the safety net of your training. Make unforgettable memories with your colleagues, attendings, hospital staff, and patients. It takes a large village and almost a decade to train one surgeon and we are honored that you chose to seek our advice to be a part of your journey into becoming a surgeon.

S. Seng (✉)
Crozer Chester Medical Center, Upland, PA, USA
e-mail: sirivan.seng@crozer.org

© The Author(s), under exclusive license to Springer Nature
Switzerland AG 2023
A. Ratnasekera et al. (eds.), *General Surgery Residency Survival Guide*,
https://doi.org/10.1007/978-3-031-25617-2_49

Index

A
ABSITE Quest, 38
Accreditation Council for Graduate Medical
    Education (ACGME), 133
ACGME case log system, 56
Adaptability, 205
Adjusted gross income (AGI), 107
American Board of Surgery (ABS), 9
American Board of Surgery Training Exam
    (ABSITE) approaches, 5, 25
    and certifying exam, 11, 12
    and qualify exam, 10, 11
    reading plan, 10
Anki, 38
Anticipation, 47
Anxiety, 201, 202
Aristotle, 79
Assigned task, 137
Attending-resident relationship, 154

B
Behind the Knife (BTK), 39
Benefits of sleep, 169
Birthdays, 97
Boot camps, 22
Bullying, 141, 142
Burnout, 179

C
Certifying exam (CE), 9
Challenge, 147, 150
Clinical mentorship, 3

Clinical teaching
    planning, 59
    residents and students, 59
    through imaging, 60
    treatment plans, 60
Coaching style leadership, 128
Collegiality, 199
Communication, 49, 75, 115
Complexity, 150
Coordinator, 30
COVID-19, 191, 193, 194
Culture, 162
Curbside consultation, medical
    liability, 65
Curriculum vitae (CV) preparation
    academic societies and
        certifications, 34
    accomplishments and experiences, 34
    education, 34
    hobbies and interests, 34
    institutional guidelines, 35
    personal information, 34
    professional connections, 33
    professional references, 34
    professional work, 34
    research, 34
    research experience, 33
    revisit and update, 33

D
Death, 115–117
Delegation, 137, 139
Difficult attending, 153, 154